Author

Russell Tregonning, an orthopaedic and knee specialist, trained in New Zealand, England and Canada. A senior consultant for over 40 years, he also lectured at Otago University medical school in Wellington, New Zealand. His passionate interest in the evolving science of knee injuries and arthroscopic and knee replacement surgery have made him a sought-after speaker to doctors and the sports medicine community. A resident of Wellington, he is an environmental activist, working with a team of medical professionals to alert the public to the dangers that the climate crisis poses to human health. His first book, *They Made Me: Granny Gridgeman and My Otago Family Pioneers*, was 2021 co-winner of the Kevin McAnulty Award of the New Zealand Society of Genealogists.

OTHER BOOKS FROM ATUANUI PRESS

Culture in a Small Country: The Arts in New Zealand by Roger Horrocks

A Book of Seeing by Roger Horrocks

On the Farm: New Zealand's Invisible Women by David Hall

A History of Queen's Redoubt and the Invasion of the Waikato by Ian Barton and Neville Ritchie

Time to Make a Song and Dance: Cultural Revolt in Auckland in the 1960s by Murray Edmond

Tomorrow the World by MK Joseph

Drongo by Ian Richards

Cocktails with Molotov and Tea with Mr Lee by Bernard Brown

The Waikato: A History of New Zealand's Greatest River by Paul Moon

Ghost South Road by Scott Hamilton

This Explains Everything by Richard von Sturmer

Emily Jackson: A Painter's Landscape edited by Bronwyn Nicholson

Re-inventing New Zealand: Essays on the Arts and the Media by Roger Horrocks

Then It Was Now Again: Selected Critical Writing by Murray Edmond

Blood and Bone:

Revelations of an Orthopaedic Surgeon

Russell Tregonning

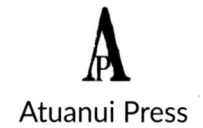

Atuanui Press

For Pamela, my rock.

First published in 2022 by Atuanui Press Ltd
1416 Kaiaua Road, Mangatangi, Pōkeno, 2473
www.atuanuipress.co.nz

Copyright © Russell Tregonning 2022
ISBN: 978-1-99-115913-7

Cover photograph by Louise Goossens

Cover design by Ellen Portch

All rights reserved.
No part of this book may be reproduced without prior permission
from the publisher, except as provided under New Zealand
copyright law.

Contents

1. **The Final List**: My last operating list – an ACL reconstruction 8
2. **Exiting the Stage**: Last operation ever – a knee replacement 24
3. **Why Medicine?**: Factors in choosing this career 41
4. **Intermediate Year**: Initiation into the first year at university 45
5. **The Real Deal**: Introduction to medical training, anatomy dissection room 51
6. **Burn Out**: Taking on too much clinical medicine and extra-curricular activities 59
7. **Clinical Realities**: Horror watching the first operation and delivering first babies 65
8. **The Nitty Gritty**: Stresses and rewards of a very junior relieving doctor 71
9. **Steep Learning Curve**: Life as a junior doctor, and choosing surgery 79
10. **The Locum Life**: GP work, sailing to UK and studies in surgical sciences in London 99
11. **Final Judgement**: Final surgical entry exams in London 111
12. **Joining the Herd**: Junior surgeon training and case studies 121

13. Going It Alone: Advocating for better work conditions and opposition.............................135
14. In Mackenzie Country: GP locum work in Twizel..149
15. Toronto Finishing School: A different surgical planet; learning new techniques......................155
16. Arthroscopy: Further revolutionary new techniques and burn-out..............................173
17. Some Doctors Eat Their Young: Difficulties finding a surgeon's job back home 180
18. Knees Up: Back on the job and early knee surgery research...................................190
19. Scope for Surgery: Kenepuru hospital – new techniques and instrumentation 204
20. Complications: Mistakes causing trauma to patient and surgeon.................................218
21. Dangerous Bacteria: Infection, an ever present threat to orthopaedic operations 234
22. Passing On the Baton: Experiences as a surgeon-teacher 250
23. A Late Awakening: Women in orthopaedics......265
24. Union Man: Challenging an abrupt dismissal......287

Acknowledgements 297

Author's Note

The clinical case reports and other historical descriptions in this book are based on real events. I have changed the names of most patients and some colleagues and at times altered details to protect the privacy of patients, colleagues and their families.

1.

The Final List

Bowen is a small private hospital in a peaceful setting among green hills. It's 2014 and I'm about to start on the first case of my last operating list. I have worked in this hospital for 30 years, adding private practice to my public hospital work. In the past nine years, I have done all my surgery here.

My patient, Gill, is twenty-two. Six months ago she tore the anterior cruciate ligament (ACL) in her knee while playing netball. Ligaments are fibrous rope-like structures attached to bone on either side of joints; they stabilise the joints by restraining unwanted movements. The ligament Gill has torn is the weaker of the two crossed (therefore 'cruciate') ligaments that prevent abnormal front-to-back and rotational movements between the two longest bones in the body, the femur and the tibia. The longer the bone the more force it can exert at the joint. The forces that this ligament must resist, particularly in sport, are huge.

My job is to reconstruct the torn ligament. New Zealand surgeons perform over 3000 such operations each year. About 80 percent of the injuries occur in sport – most often in rugby, then netball and football. I know from my own cases that they're mainly caused by the person falling awkwardly from a leap. A sudden twist is also common, particularly if the person also plants their foot and stops suddenly.

I have several times visited a fellow knee surgeon, John Bartlett, in Melbourne. One time, John took me to watch the grand final of Australian rules football at the Melbourne Cricket Ground. 'Aussie rules' is a contact sport played by two teams of 18 on an oval field. I found out why some New Zealanders refer to it as aerial ping-pong: players repeatedly propel themselves skyward. Gravity operates in Australia, so these tall lithe athletes must then hit the ground and sometimes they are out of control, particularly if they've been jostled while airborne. The game therefore provides knee surgeons with a rich harvest of ACL injuries.

John was team surgeon for Collingwood, one of the

finalists. He kept pointing to his patients – he seemed to have reconstructed the knees of about half the team. I later observed him operating. His technique involved using a strip of tendon harvested from the front of the kneecap and the tibia below. Until then I had used a technique I had learnt in Canada a decade before, taking a strip of tissue from the side of the thigh.

This tissue was weak, so I would have to harvest a long, wide strip. This left a visible scar, and in some people a bulge. Usually this could be hidden by clothing, but it was obvious when the person wore shorts. One patient told me, 'I like to show my friends my "shark bite scar".' I didn't think this did my reputation much good. I was keen to learn John's new technique, which was less disfiguring.

Some people cope quite well without a functioning ACL, particularly if they build up muscle and avoid sports that involve jumping or sudden changes in direction. However, Gill is keen on netball and can't bear the thought of giving it up. I'm completely sympathetic – when I was young, rugby and other sports played an important part in my life – but I tell her that if she continues to play netball and falls repeatedly, there is a danger of more and serious damage to many of her knee structures, and eventually permanent injury to the glassy and extremely slippery cartilage covering the bones inside her knee, a condition called post-traumatic osteoarthritis.

The Final List

Gill has choices to make. The first is whether to have surgery. If she decides on this, the second is whether to have me use tendons from the front or the back of her knee.

I explain the pros and cons of surgery. Like most patients, Gill is unsure. She poses a question I commonly have to answer: 'What would you do?' I tell her that these days I only cycle or walk for exercise so I would go for maximum muscle build-up and modify my activities. But her needs, as a young active athlete, are completely different. 'If you want to get back to netball, I recommend surgery,' I say.

Knee tendons have fibres that are predominantly linear: they are designed to transmit muscle power to bend and straighten the knee. By contrast, the anterior cruciate ligament is a beautifully complex structure of fibres of various lengths curling around each other, perfectly made for the job of restraining the movement of the knee's long bones, which can twist on each other as well as bend and straighten. Most ACL reconstructions result in a more stable knee, but the knee is never as good as the original uninjured joint. The graft may stretch with time, particularly if not implanted precisely. There may be pain in the sites where the material has been harvested, and numbness in the front of the knee, making kneeling uncomfortable.

Also, if Gill plays netball there is a chance the graft will rupture.

We discuss the different techniques. I tell her I have about the same results for each, but fewer complications with hamstring tendons from the back of the knee. Even so, tendon grafts are relatively poor replicas. Not surprisingly they can fail to give a perfect result. But not always. Recently I met 44-year-old James in my fracture clinic. He had come with a minor fracture after falling off his mountain bike. When I introduced myself, he immediately said, 'I know you – you operated on my knee 20 years ago. I went back to play basketball nine months after the operation and played intercity A-grade twice a week for eight years.'

He reminded me of his dramatic injury. 'I suddenly changed direction. There was nobody near me. My knee wobbled and collapsed – I felt as if I'd been shot.' From his scars it was obvious I'd used a patellar-tendon graft. My examination showed it was intact. The knee was stable, two decades after reconstruction. My step was light for the rest of the clinic.

For patients to qualify for surgery, they need to undertake a vigorous exercise programme. Gill tells me she's had an extensive course of physiotherapy to strengthen her leg muscles. She also bikes and swims, both ACL-friendly

The Final List

activities. But her knee is still unstable: a sudden twist or sharp movement can cause her to drop to the ground in pain. She's mystified as to how one simple fall has spelled the end of her active lifestyle. 'There was no one even near me when it happened,' she says. 'I just landed awkwardly from a leap and felt a snap in my knee. I thought I'd broken something, but the X-ray was normal. Now when I fall, it feels as if my knee goes out of joint. It swells up immediately. I can't play ping-pong, let alone netball.'

Gill's is a common story. I've heard about dramatic events like this often. When I ask, 'What do you think happened to your knee?' the patient reports a sensation of something 'breaking', 'dislocating' or 'coming apart'.

We are in the pre-op bay. I tell Gill I will mark her affected leg with a felt-tip pen. I ask her which limb is unstable. She looks startled: 'Doctor, surely you're not in doubt.' I explain I have to hear her tell me yet again, so we are absolutely certain. She laughs nervously.

I meet up with Wendy, the anaesthetist rostered onto my list. I like working with Wendy: she always imparts a reassuring warmth to both patients and me. One of the other more flamboyant anaesthetists is known to greet surgeons with, 'Hi, I'm your knock-out girl this morning.'

Wendy talks quietly with Gill, then bends down and injects a syringe of liquid into her IV line. She asks her to start counting out loud. Gill gets to six, then there is silence. She is no longer conscious.

Private patients choose their surgeon but not their anaesthetist. I've always thought this is somewhat back-to-front: the anaesthetist has the patient's life in her hands while I'm only in charge of a limb. However, modern anaesthesia is safe, particularly for elective surgery. Both Wendy and I have explained to Gill what to expect and outlined the risks of the procedure. One of Wendy's fellow anaesthetists, Andrew, likes to sum up the risks by asking the patient, 'How did you get to the hospital?' The patient almost invariably says, 'By car.' Andrew: 'Well, you've just survived the greatest hazard to your health today.'

Getting a patient safely to sleep and waking them later are demanding tasks, but during the operation, if the anaesthetic goes to plan (as it almost always does), the job is quite monotonous. I watch enviously as my anaesthetic colleagues read their journals during surgery. Very occasionally, though, if a patient's oxygen levels plummet, things get tense and busy for the anaesthetist. The situation requires great skill and concentration. There's a saying: General anaesthesia is 99 percent boredom and one percent terror. I have never seen Wendy seriously terrified.

We wheel Gill into the operating theatre. I'm feeling a bit hyper as I usually do before an operation, a mixture of excitement and slight apprehension. Gill's knee was very unstable in the clinic. I need to get this operation exactly right.

Wendy injects a large slug of antibiotic into Gill's vein to reduce the chances of infection after the operation. A deep infection, although uncommon with this type of surgery (less than one percent), can result in complete failure. We almost always have to operate again, sometimes more than once, to wash out the knee and remove infected material. Sometimes we need to take out the graft to eradicate the infection. The patient requires industrial doses of IV antibiotic and sometimes another grafting operation.

With Gill safely asleep, I perform a vital physical examination; I apply force to both knees and observe how much the bones move on each other.

The knee is the largest and most complex of the body's joints. We have an MRI of Gill's knee that shows all the structures in wonderful detail, but I need to know more. When Gill was awake, testing the stability of her knee had to be done vigorously and this could be painful. There was no point yelling, 'Relax!' as I have seen some junior doctors do. A patient may tense up even more, acting involuntarily to prevent pain.

It's only when Gill is completely relaxed like this that I can tell exactly how unstable her knee is, what ligaments are too loose and therefore what we need to correct. As I manipulate the knee I say, 'Hey team, have a look at this. This is as unstable as they get.' I partially dislocate the knee, pushing the tibia forward off the femur with a sudden internal twisting motion. This is quickly followed by a visible jerk as I stop twisting and the tibia sharply falls back into place.

This means Gill's anterior cruciate ligament is completely torn. I don't repeat this alarming disruption of the knee as I know from experience it can make the knee lining bleed, clouding the knee and making vision difficult when I later view its interior using arthroscopy, a technique for examining the inside of joints.

I perform the test on Gill's other knee. Everyone's knees have ligaments of slightly different flexibility but side-to-side differences in a patient are rarely great, so the comparison with a patient's normal knee is a valid test. Gill's other knee is within the normal range of stability.

From all the tests I judge that the only ligament torn on Gill's bad knee is the ACL. The other three main ligaments are normal.

I now try to dislocate the kneecap by pushing it from its normal position in the front of her knee to an abnormal position on the outside. My aim is to discover if she has recurrent patellar dislocation, another knee instability which, like ACL deficiency, is caused by a sudden knee twist and may repeatedly cause disabling 'drop knee'.

The Final List

If Gill were awake, she would feel a familiar and unpleasant sensation as the bone started to go out of joint. She would probably grab my arm to stop me continuing.

I can't make Gill's patella leave its shallow groove in the femur. The kneecap is stable. I now know for sure that we have only one ligament to attend to. 'Okay guys,' I say. 'Let's restring this knee.'

The main drama is about to start. I mask, scrub and glove up. We don sterile costumes. We need help as we can't tie ourselves into our gowns: it's a task for an assistant. An Eagles CD is slotted into the sound system. It's not what I'd choose at home – I'm more into classical music – but I like it well enough, and I know most of the others do too. The music puts me in a positive frame of mind and adds to a feeling of camaraderie.

I always wait until a patient is well asleep before starting the music. I'm mindful of a colleague who got into trouble for operating on the wrong leg. At the investigation into the incident, the patient reported that when she entered the theatre there was a festive atmosphere, with loud music being played. She believed the operating team were not fully concentrating. If things get complicated and stressful, I will ask for the music to be stopped to help me concentrate.

I walk over to the operating table, into the bright pool

of light beaming down on the patient, and join the scrub nurse, Megan. The dialogue begins. 'Paint brush, please.' I'm handed a gauze square held by forceps. I paint Gill's leg with chlorhexidine, an antiseptic solution. It has a red colouring agent so we know we've thoroughly covered all the skin that will need to be exposed during the operation. The skin is now a garish pink.

We place bilious green sterile drapes above and below the knee to exclude all unsterilised skin and apply sticky-based plastic cling to hold the drapes on and further seal off the skin around the area where I will make the incision. I call out, 'Handle, please.' I reach up and screw the sterile light handle into place. I manipulate it to direct the bright stream of light onto the operative field; I'll be able to adjust this during the operation, if necessary.

On the inside of the tibia, just below the knee, I cross-hatch the skin with a pen to ensure I close the wound edges precisely at the end of the operation. We elevate the gaudy pink and green leg. An assistant inflates a tourniquet high on the thigh to provide me with as bloodless a field as possible. The time is noted. We have 90 minutes before an alarm will sound, indicating we may harm the leg if we deny it blood any longer.

We move swiftly into our routine, quick and deliberate without too much haste. Like actors, we know our roles from many previous performances.

The Final List

'Knife please.' I feel confident but also a bit nostalgic. On this, my final operating list, I am remembering back to my first tentative skin incision, the sweaty feeling with my heart racing as I mentally prepared myself for the act of entering the patient's body. Would I feel faint, I wondered, as I did as a student when I first saw surgery? I was tentative. My surgeon supervisor told me to press harder to cut through skin and the fat below. It was a weird feeling and disconcerting, but the tissues parted cleanly. I felt exhilarated: now I was in control, not just a nervous spectator.

Decades doing this task have taken away the exhilaration and the anxiety. It's all routine now. I make a short incision along the middle of the cross-hatch with a quick deliberate sweep. The blood wells up.

'Burner please, Megan.' She hands me the diathermy wand. I methodically stop the bleeding, cauterising each bleeding vessel in the skin edges. The wound is now dry and I have good vision.

I harvest two hamstring tendons by cutting them off the tibia and detaching them from their muscle bellies above. I then double both tendons and fashion a single quadruple-strand graft by suturing them together. By measuring the graft's diameter, I can choose the correct sized drill to create sockets in both the femur above and the tibia below through which to feed the graft.

With a sharply pointed scalpel, I make two stab

wounds in the front of the knee. In one I insert a tube-like instrument, the canula. Through this I pass a long thin telescope, four millimetres in diameter, that contains fibre optics to illuminate the joint's interior. I attach a camera to the eyepiece; this relays a picture onto a screen.

I turn a valve on the canula to allow saline solution from an elevated bag to continuously drip into the joint. This will keep the inside clear of debris and give me clear vision. I now insert a metal probe and manipulate the structures under suspicion. We peer at the inside of Gill's knee on the screen. Her ACL has only a string of residual tissue left.

The MRI has suggested there may be a tear on the meniscus. There are two menisci in each knee, one on each side. Made of tough gristle, they act as shock-absorbers. Menisci often tear at the same time as an ACL injury, or during subsequent knee 'giving way' episodes. If necessary, we can use various cutting, biting and chewing instruments inserted into the joint through the second stab hole to trim loose pieces.

The menisci and cartilage-bearing surfaces look fine. 'Okay team,' I say, 'kill The Eagles. Let's fix this knee.'

I carefully identify the stumps of the old anterior cruciate ligament and make tunnels through which we pass the graft. We fix it to bone above and below the joint at just the right tension with screws. We have stabilised the knee, a relief for me and satisfaction for the whole team. 'Please turn the music on again,' I say.

I want Gill to have as little pain as possible when she wakes up, so I liberally inject long-acting local anaesthetic into the edges of the incision and into the back of the thigh from where I've taken the hamstrings. In the past we relied solely on powerful narcotics such as morphine to numb pain. The potential downsides were drowsiness, slow and ineffective breathing, and sometimes severe nausea and constipation. Patients occasionally received more morphine than they needed. More often they received too little because nurses feared creating an addiction.

A current technique to precisely target post-operative pain is patient-controlled analgesia. The patient is given a saline drip to which has been added morphine or a similar strong pain-relieving drug. He or she presses a button to release a dose and deaden pain. Dosages are carefully monitored so overdose is not a problem.

I always enjoy the last part of an operation: closing the wound. This is when we can depart from the script. Megan is telling Wendy about her newly acquired handbag. 'How many handbags does a woman need?' I ask Megan. 'Heaps,' she replies. 'I have handbags that fit inside handbags.'

I'm out of my depth. I change tack. 'Okay,' I say, 'let's put some legs on this centipede.' Megan hands me the staple gun. I find inordinate pleasure in making a perfectly neat closure. I want as pretty a scar as possible: it appeals to my sense of order and I love it when the patient is pleased. I carefully line up the hatch marks to join the ends. This is when I sometimes tell my nursing assistants or trainee surgeon about the successful lawsuit taken against an American surgeon who failed to get the marks joined up exactly. There's not much chance Gill will sue me, but I erase the ink marks anyway. There will be no ill effect if the skin is not closed precisely but there's no point inviting criticism.

'Let's get out of here. Mrs Brown is calling,' I say as Megan hands me an adhesive waterproof dressing, soft padding, crepe bandage and splint. 'Mrs Brown' is code for coffee. When I have patients in a waiting room, I use this term if they are in earshot. I worry that they won't like the idea of our taking a break. Here I don't have to disguise the fact: everybody wants a break before the next case as much as I do.

'Tourniquet off, please.' The cuff makes a hissing sound as the pressure releases. We finish before the alarm sounds. Act one is over.

Several hours later I take off the splint. 'Welcome back, Gill.' I say. 'How are you feeling?'

She says she has little discomfort other than a sore throat from the tube used by the anaesthetist. This is good.

The Final List

A patient who wakes in severe pain or nauseated in the early hours after surgery is primed to have a stormy recovery. I want Gill to feel able to use her leg a little without fear of pain. This will help her rehabilitation.

'Everything went really well,' I say. 'Your knee is stable again. It's safe for you to do a little exercise now. Can you brace your leg with your quads by shrugging up your kneecap? And bend your knee a little, if it's not too sore. But don't make it hurt.' Later, when the local anaesthetic has worn off, the pain will kick in, but meanwhile Gill will feel confident she can move her knee without harming it.

2.

Exiting the Stage

IT'S NOW TIME FOR MY VERY last operation. Ever. I can't quite grasp this. The drama of surgery has been my regular fix for such a long time; I'm addicted to the pleasure-enhancing substances my brain produces. I'm not going cold turkey, so my withdrawal symptoms won't be severe. For about a decade I've restricted surgery and consultations to half-day sessions. This has been different from earlier in my career when the days were long, sometimes stretching into night. I always tried to get home for dinner with my family even if I had to go back later to operate. My son Mark recently reminded me, 'Dad, you went off to work energetic and lively. I thought, he really enjoys his work.

Exiting the Stage

But in the evening I didn't ever hear you say what a good day you'd had, that an operation had gone well. You seemed tired and drained.'

In recent years, with less pressure, I've really enjoyed the work, but as with any fine skill, surgery requires constant practice. I can't just dribble on. I'm aware that two of my colleagues went on too long and got into trouble with the Medical Council right at the end of their careers.

I don't have to abandon medicine completely. I can still lecture medical students, perhaps see patients in fracture clinics. There's the possibility of doing locums or assessing patients for the Accident Compensation Commission. And I have interests outside surgery. Maybe I'll write a book?

Nevertheless, it's a weird feeling as I scrub up for the final time. I enjoy the usual banter with the nursing assistants. They are a pleasure to work with and a key part of the success of any surgery. Surgery is a team effort, with everyone playing their part in the carefully orchestrated event. I will miss this warm bonding time.

Kevin, my patient, is 71, a retired teacher who spends a lot of time helping his busy son and daughter-in-law with his grandchildren. He's troubled by an increasingly painful right knee. The pain is mainly on the inside of the knee. He experiences a chronic ache when walking and sharp, knife-like pain if he twists suddenly. The knee is waking him at night and making him grumpy. He worries that he's becoming difficult to live with. He takes maximum doses of anti-inflammatory pills and painkillers but still limps and can't walk far. He can no longer play golf, which has been his main form of exercise and a valued social contact with his friends.

He is otherwise well, making him a good candidate for surgery. 'My mate Eric has had two tin knees put in and is back golfing. His handicap has even gone down,' he says hopefully. 'Can you do that for me, doc?'

I defer. I tell him that if I thought my golf handicap would go down, I might consider having the operation myself. I can't guarantee a perfect knee, but modern knee replacement is usually successful, I say. Most patients are pleased with the pain relief and improved mobility.

I examine Kevin's knees. When he stands, his right knee is bowed compared to his left, and when he walks he has an obvious limp. There are three compartments in a knee – inside, outside and kneecap joint. I ask Kevin to lie down, then I put pressure on the outside compartment of his knee and the knee cap. This causes him no pain. When I put pressure on the inside of his knee, he yelps.

I can straighten his knee by putting pressure on the outside, so the bowing is not a fixed deformity. I test for ACL function. It's fine. When I lift Kevin's legs straight up off the bed the right knee can't fully straighten, but the deficit is slight.

Kevin's weight-bearing X-ray shows there is no space between the bones on the inside of his knee. Kevin has worn out his wonderful, near frictionless surface cartilage tissue, like a car tyre worn down to the backing. This is age-related 'wear-and-tear'.

From the X-ray of the side of Kevin's knee, I see that his ACL is probably intact. As knee osteoarthritis advances, this ligament can become crushed and tear as bone outgrowths impinge on it during motion. If Kevin decides on surgery, the integrity of the ACL will be one of the factors determining the type of knee replacement operation he will have.

Although Kevin has only moderate signs of arthritis, he has disabling pain. He has tried the gamut of conservative treatment. He has had two injections of steroid, a powerful anti-inflammatory. This helped, but only temporarily. He is starting to get indigestion from anti-inflammatory pills; stomach bleeding may be next. He has tried physiotherapy, but pain relief was also fleeting.

We discuss the pros and cons of knee replacement surgery. He is keen to go for it, and my assessment is that he is likely to benefit from it. But surgery involves risk. I encourage him to continue with the muscle exercises recommended by his physiotherapist. His prolonged disability and reduced amount of exercise have made his leg muscles weak and wasted. The stronger his leg is before surgery, the quicker will be his recovery.

The common symptoms of pain and stiffness with an arthritic knee are often intermittent at first, so it's wise to wait for the pain to become continuous and affect movement significantly before undertaking major surgery. Patients on our waiting lists sometimes get better and take themselves off the list. This means they probably shouldn't have been there in the first place. Surgery would have been too soon for them. I am comfortable advising patients to try all non-operative treatments first. Considering golf, I usually will not operate on a patient who can still play 18 holes without a cart.

I'm guided by the maxim: If in doubt, don't operate. Some patients may go away from a consultation thinking I'm a fizzer: I turn down more patients for surgery than I book. I tell them to try all the non-surgical methods first. But Kevin has long-standing continuous pain and disability, so replacement is a wise choice. He is fit to withstand the rigours of the surgery.

I spell out the main complications and give Kevin a pamphlet about them. I don't want to scare him, but I want him to be fully informed of the risks. And it is a professional requirement: if I don't inform him and he suffers a surgical complication, the Medical Council or Health and

Disability Commission may investigate and discipline me.

I offer two common types of knee replacements to patients like Kevin. One is called a partial unicompartmental replacement, or 'uni' – it replaces only half the main joint, the inside compartment. The alternative, chosen by most New Zealand orthopaedic surgeons, is a full knee replacement, or 'total'. This replaces the whole knee joint, either two or three compartments. The kneecap compartment, even if worn, is often not replaced if symptoms indicate that pain in the front of the knee is not major. Almost all replacements done in New Zealand are registered in the New Zealand Orthopaedic Association's Joint Registry. Data in 2019 showed the number of totals dwarfed unis by about nine to one.

Both uni and total have pros and cons, and surgeons debate their merits endlessly. The total involves a substantially longer incision, dislocates the whole knee joint, and may remove both cruciate ligaments. Blood loss is greater and some patients require transfusion. The hospital stay and recovery time are usually longer and the operation is more expensive.

After a total knee replacement, the risks of deep infection and the feared deep vein thrombosis, although small, are also higher. Rehabilitation is slower and knee stiffness more likely. A stiff knee is a major inconvenience and sometimes difficult to treat.

But if Kevin has a total there may be less chance he will need a further operation later on. This is why many surgeons justify the more invasive 'total' even when the osteoarthritis is confined to only one part of the knee. Data from joint registries worldwide show that the number of second operations (or 'revisions') after unis is significantly higher than after totals.

But there's a hitch. Revisions of unis are easier technically: they are more straightforward operations with less risk of complication. Hence surgeons are more inclined to revise a painful uni than an equally painful total. Comparing the success of unis versus totals by comparing revision rates is therefore like comparing apples with oranges. Interestingly, when patients are asked, those who have had a uni report less pain and better function than those who've had totals.

The uni I use was conceived and developed at Oxford University in the 1960s by two men: an orthopaedic surgeon and an engineer. John O'Connor, a lecturer in engineering science, was looking for funding for structural joint research. His field was the kind of joints you might find on an aeroplane. Confusion about his intentions led to a chance encounter with John Goodfellow, an orthopaedic surgeon and researcher at the Nuffield Orthopaedic Centre. The two men teamed up to try to solve problems with existing human knee joint replacement devices: either the surfaces wore out quickly or the components loosened and fell out, or both.

The most common cause of failure of an artificial joint is destruction of the bone to which it's attached. Tiny plastic particles are generated by friction between the artificial joint's metallic (or sometimes ceramic) parts and its plastic parts. These particles can penetrate the bone/cement or bone/metal join. The bone reacts to the foreign material by secreting substances that cause the bone to disintegrate. A layer of scar tissue forms. Being weaker than bone, this cannot stabilise the artificial joint, which then rattles around in the bone causing more destruction and pain. An X-ray will show the destroyed bone and replacement scar tissue as an irregular zone of shading surrounding the artificial joint.

The Oxford team's breakthrough was to make the plastic bearing mobile. This resulted in less wear and a fuller range of movement: the knee joint could twist as well as bend, giving patients a more natural range.

The Oxford team claimed their patients recovered twice as fast as those operated on with the standard procedure, and three times as fast as those with a total knee replacement. On top of the mechanical advantages I saw in the mobile bearing design, the minimally invasive technique for its insertion had persuaded me to make the Oxford my uni of choice for my patients.

Blood and Bone

I love the look of its smooth motion. When the knee moves, the plastic bearings slide around easily on the metal surfaces. The bearings have a minimum thickness of three millimetres, so in theory they should last 300 years. The maximum nine-millimetre-thick bearing should last nearly a millennium. Loosening of the joint due to wear should therefore be minimal.

The downside of a mobile bearing is that it can dislocate. I warn Kevin of this unusual occurrence. I show him a total and a uni – both removed during revision operations – implanted in mock plastic bones. 'Wow, the total replacement sure is heavy,' he says. 'Will I put on weight if you use this?' I tell him there will be no real weight gain as the pieces of bone I will remove, with their marrow and blood, weigh little different than the artificial joint.

He flexes the two Oxford uni metal components. 'I see what you mean about the plastic bearing gliding easily,' he says, and laughs. 'I'll be able to run faster with one of these.' I tell him surgeons don't recommend patients run on their knee replacements. It's a bit of a heavy response to his light-hearted joke, but it's useful to slip in this piece of advice.

I ask if there's anything else he wants to know. Some patients aren't curious and just want me to get on with the operation, but Kevin is not one of them. He asks, 'How long will my wound be and what kind of stitches will you use? My mate had skin staples. One of the wounds got really red and he had to get the staples removed early.'

I tell him I will use skin staples.

'But isn't the body more likely to reject metal than fine stitches?' he says.

I tell him the chances of his developing inflammation through metal staples is about the same as with nylon stitches – both are foreign materials. The Australasian College of Surgeons recommends the use of staples as there is less risk of a surgeon pricking him or herself and contracting an infection, such as hepatitis or AIDS, spread by exchange of bodily fluids. Also, I can staple his wound closed twice as fast and just as neatly. And the faster we get him awake the better.

'What will you do to help with pain after the operation?' he asks.

'Before you wake, I will inject long-acting local anaesthetic into your wound. This will work for up to six hours. After it wears off, you will be able to use your drip – just press the button and you'll get a safe dose of morphine. After that, we'll give you oral medication, strong morphine-like drugs such as codeine or Tramadol, to take at home for a short time. Later, you can use paracetamol and anti-inflammatories such as Brufen and Voltaren. I check that he doesn't have indigestion, asthma, renal trouble or other conditions that mean he can't use this medication safely.

'Will I need physio?'

'Yes,' I say. 'Physios will visit you in the hospital and show you exercises. You should keep these up at home. They may be a little painful but they won't affect the wound. If you don't try to move your knee early on, strong bands of scar tissue can bind it and cause stiffness. These are hard to break down later.'

I sense Kevin is pretty phlegmatic; he will probably exercise well and get a good range of motion. Patients who are anxious and fearful of pain can be too scared to do the required exercises. Regular confidence-building with a physiotherapist can help these patients enormously.

Kevin wants to know how long he'll be in hospital. All going well, and if his knee is suitable for a uni, about a couple of nights, I tell him. For a total, a night or two more.

'How long before I can walk the grandkids to school, about half a kilometre?'

'Perhaps three to four weeks, probably with one crutch or a stick at first.'

He now gets down to the nitty-gritty. 'How long before I can get back on to the golf course?' This question often comes first. Returning to sport is all-important for some patients, and certainly much more important than when they can return to work. 'If you can use a cart, about a month,' I say. 'Maybe six weeks if you're walking.'

And then Kevin asks an important question that all

patients considering surgery should ask of their surgeon: 'What's the success rate of knee replacements?'

I don't want him to have unreasonable expectations. Modern knee replacements mostly work well, but a knee of metal and plastic is a pale replica of the real thing, which has evolved over millions of years. A replacement can transform the life of a patient, but some artificial joints are not as good as others and patients' response to surgery varies enormously. The worse a person's symptoms are before the operation, the more pleased he or she is afterwards.

I tell Kevin that about four out of five patients are pleased or very pleased with the results of knee replacement. About 20 percent are not totally happy, and some among them are unhappy.

A question almost all patients fail to ask me is: 'How many of these operations do you do in a year and what are your results?' Even though he doesn't ask, I give Kevin my personal stats.

So far I am favouring a uni for Kevin. To be extra sure, I put pressure on the compartments of both knees as the radiographer takes more X-rays. The final test, though, will be at the beginning of the operation. When I open the knee I will need to confirm that the thick black line on the X-ray really does represent continuous, near normal cartilage. I check with Kevin: Will it be okay if I change tack and insert a total if I see unexpectedly severe disease? He agrees.

Blood and Bone

We're in theatre. Before we prep Kevin's skin, I say to Wendy, 'Weed-killer please.' She injects a slug of antibiotic. I open Kevin's knee and my assistant retracts the wound edges. I closely inspect the cartilage. As expected, I see bone-on-bone in the medial compartment. The cartilage on the outside has only minor pitting. I probe it. It looks good. I say, 'Okay guys, let's go for the uni.'

Megan expresses satisfaction. She and the others know that this operation – even done by me, a slow surgeon – will be shorter than a total. I'm pleased too as I enjoy this type of surgery. I feel a sense of pride and satisfaction achieving a knee replacement through such a small wound. But I'm a bit anxious. Am I doing the right thing by Kevin? Is that cartilage really as good as it looks? Will it last the distance? Only time will tell.

The smaller the incision the better it is for the patient – but within reason. When I was a surgical trainee doing one of my first appendicectomies, I couldn't find the appendix. I called my senior. He rushed in, grabbed the knife and doubled the size of my incision at a single stroke. This revealed the inflamed appendix, lying hidden behind the large bowel. 'Dr Tregonning,' he said sternly, 'always remember, wounds heal from side-to-side not end-to-end.' With that he left.

I had learnt a valuable lesson: if the size of the wound threatens to hinder the success of the operation by preventing adequate vision, the wound must be made longer. Do the job well and safely. Forget your pride.

Back with Kevin we create what would be a nightmare scene for an outside observer. Thankfully, there are none. First, we hammer pins into the femur and tibia to anchor the jigs that will guide the bone-cutting and reaming. There's a piercing whine from the power tools as we cut the bone. The expression 'dry as a bone' refers only to the dead. The bone of a living person is full of blood and fatty marrow. We stir up a cloud of bone dust, blood, and marrow droplets that threatens to coat our glasses and visors. My assistant adds to the cacophony with a loud gurgling noise as a sucker vacuums away the smoke of burning bone and bits of bone and body juices flying into the air.

We clean the bony surfaces, removing marrow and fat with a pulsed 'lavage' gun that delivers saline – a mixture of salt in water – like a high-pressure garden hose. The saline pools in the wound and its droplets add to the cloud.

The bone looks like honeycomb. We dab it with swabs until it resembles a beautiful white coral. This will allow maximum penetration of the semi-liquid cement that will anchor the artificial knee firmly to bone. The cement has a long-acting antibiotic that leaches slowly into the bone, another protection against the dreaded deep infection. Today most uni surgeons use joint replacements that have a roughened back side. This encourages the bone to grow into the spaces so there's no need for cement. In the seven years since I stopped operating, statistics have shown that fewer re-operations are required with this method.

Suddenly, peace descends. There's just a gentle stirring noise as the scrub nurse mixes the cement in a bowl with a plastic spatula.

After sizing Kevin's knee, I press the components, chosen to fit, onto the bones for a few minutes until the cement hardens. I test the mobile bearing for stability and make sure it moves freely. Then, after injecting local anaesthetic into the edges of the wound, I close it with skin staples.

Kevin is awake in the recovery room. I tell him we've successfully replaced his knee with a uni. 'That's great!' he says. 'I was hoping it would be a uni.' My enthusiasm for the uni has caught on.

I ask Kevin to lift his leg straight off the bed and then flex his knee to about a right angle. He does it, gingerly. He's surprised and pleased: more brain rush for me, my final hit. It's about 52 years since I started my journey in medicine. For the last decade I've restricted work to my passion – knee surgery. Gill's and Kevin's are operations I've performed many times. Today, both are very different from those I saw as an orthopaedic trainee. Back then, both ACL rupture and knee osteoarthritis were poorly understood.

Recently, I've become less tolerant of the uncertainty inherent in performing surgery and more anxious when things don't go exactly as planned. Sometimes, if the going gets hard or I'm not certain of the best way forward, I can barely stand the inner tension. If I can't quite get the tendon graft around the corner at the back of the knee, or the prosthesis won't fit and I can't see why, I feel my chest tighten and my agitation rising. It's a huge effort to stay in control.

I silently scream: How the hell are you going to get this bloody thing in? I sometimes stamp my foot like a child; it seems better than yelling obscenities or throwing instruments. I remember a knife skidding across the floor towards me when I was a student cowering in the corner of an operating theatre. An elderly surgeon had lost his cool during a tricky part of an operation. Nobody copped the knife, but the atmosphere was electric.

I know this tension is going to continue: much-practised operations will not always go perfectly. I don't want to have a colleague tap me on the shoulder and suggest I consider retiring. I want to make that decision myself. I've asked our practice manager not to book any more surgery cases. I feel mainly relief. It's taken a while for me to come to the decision to stop operating but I'm 69.

I want out before I hit 70.

I think back to my decision to make orthopaedic surgery my career. Surgery has been a roller coaster, greatly rewarding but at times stressful. Overall, I've loved the job and I think it's suited me. Now it's time to put the knife away. For me, the drama of surgery is over.

3.

Why Medicine?

AT PRIMARY SCHOOL, AGED ABOUT TEN, I was asked what I wanted to be when I grew up. With the certainty of youth, I firmly pronounced, 'A doctor.'

I wonder why I was so sure. The earlier portents were unfavourable. My younger brother, Bruce, was born with multiple abnormalities of hands and lower limbs. The Dunedin Hospital orthopaedic clinic put on plaster casts to realign his feet. These had to be regularly changed as he grew. I was about four when I first went with my mother and Bruce into the hospital's forbidding bowels. Just getting to the clinic was scary. Hot water pipes running over our heads clanked in the cave-like corridors, making a noise a surgeon once described as 'discordant rumbles, gurgles and crackles reminiscent of machine-gun fire'.

Worse was to come. In the clinic the nurse picked up a circular saw and turned on a switch. There was a screeching whine as it roared into life. I was terrified. Was Bruce's leg going to be cut off? Bruce and my mother seemed completely calm as I panicked and wailed. Unknown to me, a plaster saw was different from an amputation saw. The circular blade merely oscillated, the vibrations making a cut in the rigid plaster-of-Paris cylinder. Bruce's leg stayed where it was.

Although I have vivid memories of this formative experience, it was just the start. The whole hospital gave me heebie-jeebies. The ground-floor corridors were windowless, and our voices echoed off the walls. Everything was unnaturally clean and shiny and there was a strong smell of antiseptic. I wanted out of there. And I didn't want to return.

My mother, Hope, was a trained nurse so it might have been her influence that overcame any doubts I had about a medical career; she often spoke about her colleagues, and always in a complimentary way. Perhaps her respect for doctors rubbed off on my older brother Garnet and me. We both became surgeons. Our sister Megan became a nurse.

Hope was the third oldest of eight children. Although

Why Medicine?

dux of her primary school, she had been taken out of secondary school early to help care for her younger siblings. She wanted to be a nurse but had not gained matriculation. Her saviour was her mother's cousin James Renfrew White. Always known as Eefie, White was a prominent Dunedin orthopaedic surgeon and a lecturer at the medical school. He was an energetic teacher and a local character, known for swinging around lamp posts and jumping over rubbish tins on his way to and from the medical school. He had many interests – literature, music, education, child welfare and physical education – and wrote and published numerous books, papers and articles. His influence within the medical establishment was considerable. He persuaded the nursing powers to let my mother into nursing school. She thrived and passed her exams easily.

In the late 1950s, children perceived as academically able were destined for a 'classical' education. At King's High School, which I attended, this included Latin and French. By the time I applied for medical school in the 1960s knowledge of Latin was no longer a prerequisite, but my grounding in it proved useful as the names in anatomy were, and still are, largely rendered in Latin.

In my final school year we were offered vocational guidance. The adviser looked through my school record. Although I had been streamed into top classes, I was not a stellar student. However, I had been conscientious and gained some honourable mentions. I was also sporty, a trait highly regarded at boys' schools. I could sprint quickly and had become senior athletic champion. Although my ball-handling ability was only moderate, I had been made captain of the First XV, possibly because the coach knew me well. He doubled as the school's music teacher and I had performed in operettas, madrigal singing and the school orchestra.

My vocational guidance master's advice was: 'You can do anything you put your mind to.' This was reassuring but I was still not 100 percent sure medicine was for me. Nonetheless, I headed to Otago University for 'intermediate' year. My academic performance there would determine whether I got into medical school.

4.

Intermediate Year

In 1963 Dunedin was the only medical school in the country. Entry was decided solely on the marks you got in written exams at the end of the intermediate year. The thinking among the medical school gatekeepers was that those with high academic marks had shown an ability to complete the demanding course (which depended on cramming then regurgitating facts). For all they knew we could have a major personality defect, a problem communicating or even a criminal record – there was no police check.

The policy tended to reward those who had had advantages in their high school education. Today, good academic grades alone are not considered sufficient to equip a doctor for the expectations of the community, including in matters of race, gender, urban versus rural background, and social equity.

In the 1960s, tertiary education was cheap for those who had passed the university entrance exam. Our fees were paid by the government and we were given expense allowances: I received £40 for the first year and £60 for second, the equivalent of about $2500 and $3750 today. I lived at home in Macandrew Bay; the medical school was only 12 kilometres away, a 20-minute ride on my motorbike.

The intermediate year comprised chemistry, physics and zoology. I was determined to pass well enough to not have to repeat it. I had none of the diversions of fellow students who lived in halls of residence or student flats. I valued the peace and quiet in which to study but felt slightly envious of the fun I was missing out on.

At lectures I thought I would be among adults. It quickly became apparent this was not the case. When a lecturer's back was turned, my bored classmates would launch paper darts from high tiers of the lecture theatre. Lecturers' attempts at humour were greeted with the stamping of feet. I felt sorry for the poor devils, but we had already learned much of the material at high school.

Intermediate Year

My parents were broadminded. There was no curfew, and I was able to experiment with alcohol, wildish parties and women. I had not drunk alcohol before. I started off slowly, occasionally riding my motorbike into town for a night of socialising with classmates at the Bowling Green Hotel, aka the BG, Bowler, or sometimes the 'green lecture theatre'.

Pubs officially closed at six o'clock. Men (I didn't ever see a woman) came straight from work, lined up jugs of beer and chugged them down: the notorious six o'clock swill. Students preferred to drink after hours. Our carefully rehearsed drill involved creeping up to the Bowling Green and surreptitiously knocking on the front door. Dot, the proprietor, would open the door a crack. Without speaking or looking at us she would scan the street, first left, then slowly right. If it was all clear we'd be ushered in with, 'Hurry boys! Now, if the sergeant bursts in – you, over there behind that door; you, behind those kegs.'

We would settle in, slightly on edge, which just gave our drinking an extra frisson. I'm not sure how our careers might have unfolded if we were caught; we didn't give that much thought.

I looked forward to my first woolstore hop. On the face of it, these events in south Dunedin warehouses were an exciting prospect. As new students we heard much about the debauchery-ridden winter rituals, where bales of wool around the dance area gave privacy and soft surfaces for assignations. Disappointingly, the stories of rampant sex were exaggerated. Dunedin has a convincing winter, and the huge barn-like spaces were frigid and unappealing. There was no furniture. Music volume routinely trumped quality and chatting up women was near impossible because of the din. On top of this, I was painfully shy.

Drinking and driving by motorcyclists was not policed. I used to ride home after student parties along the winding, unlit peninsula road. About three o'clock one freezing winter morning my motorbike lights failed. The road was slippery with ice. Alcohol-affected and navigating by instinct I somehow made it home. I cut the engine 50 metres from home, pushed the bike, opened the garage doors very quietly (they were immediately below my parents' bedroom) and tiptoed undetected into the house.

Wine-drinking was practically unheard of. Most wine was imported and beyond our means. Fortunately, the benches in our chemistry lab boasted an array of reagents, including one that was useful for organisers of student parties. One hundred percent ethyl alcohol (200 proof), mixed with orange juice, made an acceptable fruit punch. Partway through the year, the authorities wised up and the large bottles were removed from the lab benches. Many students blamed this for parties all around town being canned. More likely, the threat of the impending exams had sobered up the north Dunedin student body.

The fruit punch had been a refreshing change from the ubiquitous Speight's. Local folklore had it that this was swamp water, kept until fermented, then bottled and sold as beer. Later I worked in a holiday job at Speight's brewery. The swamp water was an urban myth: the beer was bona fide. At first, we holiday workers followed the full-timers and drank it at morning and afternoon tea, as well as at lunch time. We soon tired of this: our work needed at least a modicum of brain power. Some of the permanent workers didn't tire of it. The place was a haven for alcoholics. They fought for the quality control job, where you sat checking as bottles went past on a conveyor belt. It was easy to put a bottle down beside you as you worked and have a few swigs when the boss wasn't watching.

Continuous assessment had not yet been invented. Exams were everything. Most students played hard during the first two terms, then swotted like mad in the final weeks. In my fifth year I flatted with a friend who took this to extremes. On the night before our exam in public health, our other flatmate and I were off to bed when we saw Donald sorting his lecture notes on the floor of his bedroom. He was going to read through them before the exam started at nine next morning. Staying up all night, he annoyingly got better marks than either of us. His logic was impeccable

– cramming the year's work in one night meant there was not enough time for him to forget what he'd read.

In the vital exams at the end of the intermediate year I was anxious about physics, my weakest subject. I managed to scrape a B pass. Along with two As, this was enough to gain me entry to medical school.

5.

The Real Deal

The medical school at Otago University is about a kilometre from the main campus. As medical students we were not only physically distant from other students, we dressed differently. While the rest of the student body swanned around in jeans, T-shirts and duffle coats, we aspiring male doctors donned a collar and tie and jacket.

On entry to medical school we started five academic terms, cramming facts about the anatomy, biochemistry and physiology of the human body. From the founding of Otago Medical School in 1875, human anatomy had been the mainstay of medical education. Studying it was a shock at first. As well as lectures, we had long periods of dissection in the cadaver room. We entered the room looking like ill-dressed shop assistants in short white coats with incongruously long sleeves. There was a strong smell of formalin. The dead were lined up on metal tables. I had not seen a dead body before. Most were disturbingly emaciated.

Small groups, arranged alphabetically, were assigned a body. Each group would keep 'their' body for the next year and two-thirds. After instruction from the demonstrator, we took up a scalpel and cut into the yellowish, leathery, formalin-stained skin; the bodies had been prepared by the injection of this preservative into the blood vessels. They had rigor mortis – the joints were stiff and the tissues lacked the pliability of living tissues. There was no bleeding.

We rotated roles, one person reading aloud the anatomy text and another exposing the described structures under the skin with a knife and forceps. We dissected the muscles, nerves, blood vessels and organs to reveal their position, their extent and how they related to each other. We put the bits of removed flesh into a bucket at the end of the table.

At first, the dissecting of human flesh felt strange and nerve-wracking. I found I had little skill compared with some of my more dexterous colleagues. I was fearful of cutting vital structures. (This would become a lifelong fear.)

The Real Deal

I had no thought that my final career choice would be surgery. I would have been repelled by the very idea.

As time went on, I felt more at ease in the cadaver room. We spent long hours close to each other. We talked and joked. I became close friends with some fellow students whose surnames, like mine, started near the end of the alphabet. After a few weeks the process became routine, at times even a bit boring. Sometimes I would drift over to a friend's body to see how things were going. Usually, I wasn't so much seeking enlightenment about the mysteries of the human body as wanting to find out what parties were on that weekend or discussing the latest footy scores.

Much later, as a surgeon researching knee ligament injuries at Wellington Hospital, I would go to the morgue and dissect fresh bodies, cutting knee ligaments in sequence to work out the cause of various weaknesses caused by injury; I would then practise operations to correct them. Cutting human flesh was by then a routine experience. The morgue attendants played loud music in a tasteless, almost festive atmosphere – their way of coping with the macabre.

In a poignant poem, my classmate Rae Varcoe, today an accomplished poet, has described her feelings about her group's body.

Blood and Bone

Cadaver Spoken Here

In the beginning were the words
(artery, arcuate, acetabulum)
and the words were pared from flesh
which had dwelt among us

Adolescent and absurd
in greasy short white coats
we sliced and sawed
from axilla (a truncated space
bounded anteriorally by…)
down ligament, nerve and tendon
through anatomical space
into language

He was old and frowning
(orbicularis oculis, levator palpebrae)

His clenched hands
resisted dissection

In his dying what did they grasp?

Were terror, hope, yearning
audible over

The Real Deal

arrest, arrhythmia, asystole?

Aged man, flayed man
generous man
why did we never think
to thank you?

The greasy white coats were not the only soiled clothing. One night, sitting down to dinner at home after a dissecting session, I became aware of a strong familiar smell. The sleeves of my shirt had protruded below the sleeves of my white coat and were smeared with human fat and formalin. Luckily, I had gained complete immunity: my appetite didn't suffer.

Our professor of anatomy was a well organised lecturer and I still vividly remember his beautiful diagrams on the blackboard. He had the sort of dry wit that would not be seen as acceptable today. He said of the anatomy of the vagina, for example: 'The vagina is a fibro-muscular tube pointing downwards and forwards, or upwards and backwards, depending on your point of view.'

He was strict, fierce and appeared to have eyes in the back of his head. I discovered this the morning my motorbike skidded on ice on my way to school and I had to slow down to walking pace. When I got to the medical school,

I was late. I quietly pushed open the door of the packed theatre. (There was no back entrance.) The professor was drawing on the blackboard with his back to me. I thought I was safe but as I was about to ease down into my seat, he hollered, 'You're late! Don't bother coming into my lecture next time.' I was never late again.

Oral tests in anatomy were stressful. In one, the examiner showed me a histology slide of a cross section of tissue. I peered through the microscope. 'Describe what you see and tell me what the structure is,' he said.

Panic stations – I hadn't ever seen tissue like this. There was a clear linear layer on top of a layer of the sort of cells of which skin and the lining of various body cavities is composed. My addled brain could not work out what the clear layer was. Then I had a brainwave. 'Vaginal epithelium,' I blurted out.

'Hmmm. Very horny vagina, Mr Tregonning, don't you think? No, it's a fingernail.'

On weekdays I had a routine: ride my motorbike home after lectures; eat dinner (always cooked by my mother); spend the evening reading notes from the day's lectures, sometimes adding information from the prescribed textbook. We lived in a small house. My brothers and I studied propped up on our beds, taking turns to get up and change the LP on the stereogram. In breaks between terms,

The Real Deal

I worked in a variety of jobs that paid enough money to allow me to transport and clothe myself and buy my own beer for parties. My parents didn't ask me to pay board. I did the dishes and helped a bit around the section, but otherwise led a charmed life.

In my third year, I put extracurricular activities partially on hold to increase my chances of passing the vital first professional exam. I stopped playing first-grade rugby and switched to 'med boozers', a team of medical-school mates who rolled up on Saturdays to play in a lower grade. Afterwards in the pub we would network about where the action was that night and later join the hordes of fellow students canvassing the neighbourhood for good parties. We seldom found one. If we did, the flats were often so crowded we couldn't get in the door or, having done so, couldn't move. Then it was on to the next.

By now I had sat exams for a decade and a half, but I still felt nervous. Written anatomy exams were particularly gruelling. The questions were brutally short and the answers relied on regurgitation of facts learnt by rote. This was a test of recall rather than intelligence and there was no room for creativity. We were required to write notes about anatomical structures to include, say for a muscle, tendon attachments, general characteristics (shape and function), blood and nerve supply, and relationships to adjacent structures.

Blood and Bone

In our first professional exam, one of the questions was: 'Describe biceps brachii' (the biceps muscle in the arm). A friend made the classic mistake of not reading the question properly and wrote for half an hour on biceps femoris, a hamstring muscle on the back of the leg. His lapse was punished severely. He failed the whole multi-question exam, had to study over the Christmas holidays and return from Auckland to Dunedin early the next year to sit a 'special', another full-length exam.

I scraped into anatomy with a C. I felt as comfortable with my knowledge of anatomy as I did with physiology and biochemistry, where I had achieved distinction. This confirmed for me the vagaries of the exam process and the part played by luck. But the important thing was I had passed the first professional.

6.

Burnout

As I began fourth-year medical school, everything pointed to a more relaxing and stimulating time. The rigours of the preclinical years were over. We would now be learning about diseases and drugs, and how to question, examine and treat patients. There would be no exams for four terms. I wasn't to know that the year would turn into a nightmare. I took on more outside activities than I could manage. I began sleeping badly and waking early, feeling stressed, anxious and depressed. Although I managed to stay the course at medical school, I sought treatment from a psychiatrist and took antidepressant drugs.

In retrospect, I had shown signs at high school of

pushing myself too hard. One of my teachers, Reg Graham, had warned me not to overreach. Reg directed our school dramas. After evening rehearsals, when the buses had stopped running, he would drive me home. One night he said, 'Russell, you may be taking on too much. You need to slow down.' But I liked being busy. I thought nothing of it and changed nothing. It turned out that he could see what I couldn't.

Early in the year I was elected class representative on the Medical Students' Association. I then took on a role helping organise Easter Tournament, a New Zealand-wide inter-university multisport competition being held that year in Dunedin. In May I rehearsed vigorously for several acting roles and for singing in a sextet in the capping concert, the annual Otago University revue. Come winter I was selected in a squad to represent Otago senior rugby; we practised in the evening, often under floodlights. And I enjoyed ski trips to the mountains of Central Otago.

I began to have difficulty juggling all the balls in the air. One weekend I was to be a reserve in the Otago squad to play Southland. Sitting on the bench in those days meant no game unless you replaced an injured player, a rare event. I had an opportunity to go skiing instead with my girlfriend Pamela and sleep beside her in the university ski lodge. (No hanky-panky as we slept on communal benches; we were virgins anyway.)

Burnout

I was still stinging from being relegated to the bench when Otago played the touring Lions. I had been chosen to play, but at the last minute the regular winger had made a miraculous recovery from illness, the score that night: Otago 17, British and Irish Lions 9. Sit huddled on a bench at Invercargill's freezing Rugby Park or travel to sunny Queenstown and join Pamela skiing? It was only briefly a dilemma.

The Otago coach was not impressed. 'Tregonning, you're not a bad winger but your heart's not in it.' He got that right. I was not selected for the senior Otago reps again.

Not content with the existing diversions from study, I added the role of sports representative on the Otago University Students' Association executive. I began to find it harder and harder to concentrate on my studies and worried I might fail. After seeking medical advice, I resigned my role on the association. I felt a mixture of guilt and humiliation tempered with relief. My predominant feeling was shame: I'd let the side down. The headline in *Critic*, the student newspaper, shouted: 'Tregonning out after two weeks.' I was quoted saying, 'I'm afraid I took on the exec job without realising the vast amount of work a portfolio involves.'

I had met with Paddy Finnigan, the students' association president, to explain my predicament. Paddy was sympathetic. He told *Critic*, 'If a guy commits himself and then finds his work is likely to suffer, he is right to consider what is his highest duty.' I was grateful for his support.

In 1985, I would admire Paddy even more when he joined fellow lawyer Philip Recordon to take the New Zealand Rugby Football Union to court over the proposed All Black tour of South Africa. The 1981 Springbok tour of New Zealand had divided the country; there had been violence at the games and mass protest on the streets, the largest civil disturbance since the 1951 waterfront dispute. Paddy and Philip argued that the NZRFU was in breach of its constitution, which charged it to 'promote, foster, and develop the game'. They gained an injunction and the tour was cancelled. Paddy received death threats. The decision has been described as a New Zealand legal landmark.

Earlier I had written to Ces Blazey, the chair of the NZRFU, asking him to stop the tour. I told him I had served on the medical panel of the Wellington Rugby Football Union and had represented Otago. I expressed my fear that the tour would harm the game. I didn't get a reply. Blazey lived just down the road from my home. I regularly passed his house. I resisted the temptation to kick his white picket fence.

I was gratified to hear from a Wellington lawyer that my letter had been produced at the court case. I doubt it had any great effect, but I felt that maybe I had helped

Burnout

Paddy in a small way in return for his easing my pain 15 years before. The experience also taught me that, while speaking out may at the time feel useless, it can have an effect. This insight has driven my advocacy work. I have been a member of many protest organisations. My name is probably on a list of agitators held by the New Zealand security service.

I probably first made the list in 1981, when I boycotted the Springbok v All Blacks game in Wellington. I was to serve on the medical panel at the ground, but instead made myself available for injured players and protesters in the emergency department at Wellington Hospital. I hoped Pamela would not be brought in. She was protesting outside Athletic Park, wearing my motorbike helmet to protect herself from the police's notorious long batons.

I was not alone in finding the fourth year at medical school a difficult time: my best friend at the school, Alastair, was also suffering. Alastair was a bright student and an accomplished all-rounder. Dux of his secondary school, he had flown into medical school. He also wrote lovely poems and read widely.

I had got to know him when we worked together in the cadaver room. He constantly amazed me, effortlessly remembering anatomy texts that I laboured to learn. He was conflicted about studying medicine rather than arts.

We often listened to classical music and shared our favourite works; he introduced me to a beautiful piece of music, *Symphonie Fantastique* by Hector Berlioz.

He was a keen tramper in the South Island mountains, stimulating my lifelong love of tramping. In the first week of the May holiday break we tramped together in the Wilkin Valley. Alastair was unusually quiet but so was I: we were both stressed. When I returned to work at the hospital at the end of the holidays, I was shocked to find him there as a patient. He was recovering from a suicide attempt.

With psychiatric treatment he seemed to improve. When he was released from hospital, we met to talk and go to a film. It was to be the last time. A couple of weeks later, on November 10, 1966, the day before our second professional exams, he hired a .303 rifle, drove in his van to an isolated spot outside Dunedin, and shot himself. He was twenty-one. He left me two of his prized possessions, his Mountain Mule tramping pack and the tramping bible *Moir's Guide Book, Southern Section: Trampers' Guide to the Southern Lakes*. I didn't want them. I wanted him back.

7.

Clinical Realities

IN 1967, I LEFT HOME AND MOVED into a student flat with three male friends. An edict from the Otago University authorities had warned that unmarried male and female students should not live together. This became a contentious issue. The poet James K. Baxter, holder of the university's Robert Burns Fellowship, composed 'A Small Ode on Mixed Flatting', which contained the lines: 'The students who go double-flatting / With their she-catting and tom-catting / Won't ever get a pass in Latin; / The moral mainstay of the nation / Is careful, private masturbation.'

Meanwhile, we medical students began to have greater contact with patients. This included our first experiences in the operating theatre and the maternity suite. 'Theatre' was an accurate description of the place in which I saw my first operation. The tiered operating room at Dunedin Hospital was right across the road from the medical school. Large groups of students in a non-sterile area above the operating space would watch surgeons perform. We were not required to wear gowns or masks. Nowadays there is no tiered seating above operating theatres, operating room spaces are all kept sterile, and movement of people in and out is strictly controlled.

Sitting to look down at my first operation I was nervous. It was all very well watching and performing dissection on bloodless cadavers, but I knew this would be different and possibly scary: the surgeon we were about to watch was nicknamed 'Slasher Simpson'.

The surgery was on the leg of a patient with varicose veins. This condition involves veins in a leg becoming twisted and swollen, and occurs when the ageing valves in the veins become damaged. When you're standing, one-way valves direct blood towards your heart against gravity. When you're walking, blood is pumped upwards by the contraction of muscles. If the valves aren't working well, the veins blow out into blood-filled sacs.

Even before Simpson picked up his knife, I was worried about what we might see. We were told the largest vein in the leg was to be 'stripped'. Although I wasn't certain

Clinical Realties

what this meant, I couldn't imagine it would be anything but bloody. My suspicions were correct. It was worse than I'd imagined. After painting the patient's leg with iodine and draping the body, leaving only the leg exposed, Simpson quickly made incisions on the inside of the ankle and in the groin. Some rapid dissection revealed the top and bottom of the vein.

So far so good. There was very little bleeding as small vessels were tied off or cauterised. But then the nurse assistant handed Simpson a long wire like a piano string with a metallic ball on the end. It looked like the kind of thing you might use for garrotting. What on earth was he going to do with this medieval-looking device? I was feeling alternately hot and cold.

Simpson fed the free end of the wire into a cut in the end of the vein at the ankle and fed it right up its length to exit through an incision at the groin. Then all hell broke loose. He grabbed the top of the wire and yanked it forcibly northwards. The ball caught the vein below. As the wire was dragged upwards, it took the whole vein with it, ripping off the tributaries as it went. Blood spurted high into the air. I only just managed to get out of the theatre in time to self-administer head-down treatment.

Another discipline we had to learn about was general anaesthesia. Ether had been one of the mainstays since the mid-1800s. The others were nitrous oxide and chloroform, the latter having been abandoned in the early 1900s when it was found to cause liver and kidney damage. Ether was still being used in 1967 but it was being phased out: not only could it cause nausea and other unpleasant side effects but, being flammable, it could ignite fires in operating rooms.

We were shown how ether was administered. The device was like a fencing grill but with a more open, widely perforated mesh frame, a bit like a Hannibal Lecter mask. Over this the anaesthetist folded a gauze pad to cover the patient's face. The liquid ether was dropped onto the pad, where it vaporised and was inhaled by the patient.

We observed a junior doctor learning anaesthetic technique in order to painlessly manipulate a patient's dislocated shoulder. As the anaesthesia progressed, the doctor seemed to be having trouble getting the patient asleep. There was an air of barely controlled panic as the patient writhed about. A senior doctor rushed in to perform an emergency technique, scattering us boggle-eyed students like a flock of sparrows.

This experience was another black mark against surgery as a career. I also excluded obstetrics. As fifth-year medical students we had live-in experience in Queen Mary Hospital, where we were familiarised with the miracle of childbirth. I started to learn there, and confirmed with other experiences soon afterwards, that I would be leaving the supervision of this particular miracle in the hands of others.

We were on call for any birth, day or night. I'm not sure whether the mothers were given a choice about having students involved – I suspect not. Sometimes, when the progress of the final stage of the birth was slow and the baby's head could not be readily delivered, the birth attendant would perform an episiotomy. This is a cut made in a woman's soft tissues (the perineum) at an angle to enlarge the vulval opening. The aim is to prevent an uncontrolled tear, which might extend directly backwards into the anal sphincter, the muscle controlling faecal continence. We were taught that episiotomy wounds, correctly performed and repaired, mostly healed well.

It was one thing to accept the wisdom of the procedure, but performing it was another. The first time I had to do it was at Queen Mary Hospital, during my first delivery. The mother was screaming in pain. The midwife was yelling encouragement, demanding she push harder. The attending doctor was urging me to move fast.

Sweating, in a barely controlled panic, I picked up large surgical scissors and cut the full thickness of the perineum. I underestimated the strength of grip needed. The scissors didn't go the whole way, so I had to reopen the instrument, grip and cut harder. There was an awful crunching sensation as the taut tissues parted. I could now safely deliver the baby's head. The rest of its body followed in a torrent of fluid and blood. I grabbed the baby. It was covered in goat's cheese-like material, the vernix caseosa, the skin's protective layer. My hands were shaking. The baby was slippery. I was terrified I would drop it.

Despite culminating in the joy of the mother and the relief of the medical staff at a successful result, the act of childbirth struck me as intense, violent and potentially dangerous. If doctors weren't doing caesarean sections for the most difficult births, we were cutting and scarring women's vulvas. Clearly human evolution hadn't kept up. Our large brains need an inordinately big skull and the dimensions of the birth canal have not kept pace. My family history was littered with maternal deaths. Obstetrics as a potential career? Maybe if I could come back in a thousand years when female anatomy had evolved. But in the mid-20th century, it was not for me.

8.

The Nitty-Gritty

'House surgeon' was the long-established name for a rookie doctor working in any specialty, not necessarily surgery, in the first or second year after graduation. At the end of the fifth year we students were able to work as *acting* house surgeons while a hospital's permanent junior staff went on leave. I chose Tauranga. My flatmate and other friends were going there and the Bay of Plenty was renowned for summer sun and sizzling beaches. It seemed perfect. And at last I would have a real job – especially important as Pamela and I had recently become engaged and in anticipation I had asked and received a hospital flat for married doctors.

Blood and Bone

I was excited but very green. I hadn't appreciated what the term 'baptism by fire' meant. Tauranga Hospital, being relatively small, had few registrars – experienced doctors middling in seniority between junior house surgeons and consultants. Most of the time the only doctor available to give advice and hold my hand was a consultant.

Looking back, I regret the pain I caused the stoical patients on whom I practised. One technique was the insertion of a cannula into a vein in order to run fluid with dissolved chemicals, blood volume expanders, blood cells or whole blood into a patient, the so-called 'setting up a drip'. I felt at the time that I was the drip being set up. I was shown the technique once or twice, then left to do the next one on my own.

The favoured veins for cannulation are those just under the skin around the front of the elbow and forearm, or the back of the hand. Some of these veins are highly mobile. Many patients requiring a drip are elderly people with little subcutaneous fat, so their veins are even less fixed. Ill-fixed veins have an annoying tendency to move out of the way when they see a sharp needle coming, and when stabbed multiple times by a learner they tend to constrict.

The seasoned operator has learnt how to cope with this, but I didn't have a clue. In Dunedin, some of my classmates had spent extra time outside class visiting inpatient wards or the emergency department. While I was

The Nitty-Gritty

busy practising rugby or drama or drinking at the Bowling Green, these conscientious students were picking up the basics.

There is a saying about learning techniques in clinical medicine: 'See one, do one, teach one.' Just as with building, plumbing and other trades, surgery is an apprenticeship system. The very start of this lifelong learning of practical skills happened for me at Tauranga Hospital. And it was there that I was involved in another medical procedure in which I screwed up badly.

Before graduating, we were required to pass obstetrics by delivering a total of 20 babies. My stint at Tauranga Hospital was the last opportunity I had to make up my numbers. Shortly after I arrived I checked in at the maternity annex, described my need to carry out deliveries, and asked the midwives to call me if there were suitable uncomplicated cases.

On a hot summer's day the call came. 'Come quickly, the head is on the perineum!' This meant the baby's head had mainly passed through the bony pelvis and was starting to push against the soft tissues at the end of the birth canal. My pulse rate skyrocketed: I hadn't delivered a baby for months. I dropped what I was doing and sprinted the 100 metres to the annex. Sweating profusely, partly from exercise, partly from apprehension, I set about my work.

The delivery was easy – the baby entered the world with minimal help on my part. As I waited for the placenta I began to feel light-headed. I did some tiptoe raises to pump blood up to my head. They didn't help. I mumbled to the maternity nurse, 'I'm not feeling too good.'

I woke up in a side room. The chief midwife said, 'When you dropped to the floor, we had to drag you out here to make room for me to deliver the placenta.' I had had to leave a varicose vein operation early. Now this. I passed obstetrics and gynaecology with a B. I had delivered only 16 babies and 15 placentas.

Another job was soon to join the reject list: psychiatry. I had not been attracted to this specialty when I was a patient myself, and an experience at Tauranga Hospital confirmed this instinct.

The patient I had to admit to the psych ward was big and aggressive. He towered over me, full of rage. When I first met an adult patient, I didn't usually address them by their first name, but under the circumstances it seemed wise. I said with great respect, my voice tightening, 'Excuse me, Wayne, do you mind, I think it's better that we talk in the nurses' office here.' Behind the closed door, we sat opposite each other. I started to interview him, speaking softly and kindly to calm him down. He was agitated and believed he was being attacked. He was talking to himself and blaming the world. It was clear he was suffering from paranoid schizophrenia.

Soon, things turned nasty. We doctors were to blame, he shouted. I reached for the phone to call my senior. This galvanised him into action. 'If you use that phone or try and leave this room I'll kill you.' He looked as though he meant it.

In a flash of inspiration, I reached into my pocket and offered him a cigarette. The cigarette nearly snapped as I shakily pulled it out of the packet. He took it and I lit it for him, hoping he would now see me as a friend. I tried to chat amicably. Then I managed to divert his attention long enough to rush out the door into the ward.

Help was at hand. The police had turned up, alerted by the chief nurse. Even more important, a colleague was waiting close by with a syringe of chlorpromazine, an anti-psychotic and tranquilliser.

The man made a run for it. I was quickly out of the blocks, syringe in hand. An old rugby adage sprang to mind: 'The bigger they are, the harder they fall.' Using my best tackling technique, I brought him down and stabbed the full dose of chlorpromazine through his trousers into his buttock. Although we had not been taught the trans-trouser injection at medical school, it worked. As the policemen held him he calmed down.

Blood and Bone

Soon after this I was assigned to assist a general surgeon. Remembering my horror watching my first varicose vein operation and my recent humiliating faint in the delivery suite, I felt nervous but things went well. Doing rather than watching was the key. There was no time to think about the disturbing act of cutting through intact skin and layers of tissue. When blood spurted up, I calmly swabbed it and applied suction. My blood stayed firmly inside my skull in the correct amount. I remained warm and upright.

This was my first experience of helping at an operation. Others followed. I began to relish the cooperative atmosphere in the theatre as everyone went about their tasks with calm efficiency. (I was to learn later that this was very different from cases where emergency resuscitation and urgent surgery were needed for acute, severely injured patients. In these cases speed was of the essence, emotions were on high alert and activity could be chaotic.)

As we masked, scrubbed up and donned gowns and gloves we looked out at the panoramic view of Mount Maunganui rising from the harbour and chatted. I felt exhilarated at being part of the team. There was an air of cheerful confidence as we performed the routines to ensure patient sterility: the careful antiseptic skin painting, the placing of sterile drapes. The large overhead operating light was adjusted to shine directly on the area for incision. In those days, before sterile handles were available for one

The Nitty-Gritty

of the surgical team to screw into the light, the unscrubbed anaesthetist performed the task. I learnt an in-joke: a surgeon in first class asks the flight attendant to put out a request over the plane's PA system: 'Would the anaesthetist in economy seat 23A please come up to first class. A surgeon in 6B needs his reading light adjusted.'

Harry Watts, the surgeon, was adept. He worked with little apparent effort, seemingly in no hurry, yet the operation progressed quickly. Each member of the team knew exactly what was required. There was relaxed banter among surgeon, anaesthetist and nurses. Many years later, an outsider came into my operating theatre for a maintenance job. He'd never seen an operation before. His comments made me remember my impressions at Tauranga. He was impressed by the smooth coordination of the actors. It's no wonder so many television shows are set in hospitals, even if they are often less about the surgery than steaming love affairs among the staff.

At the end of his operations Watts would allow me to sew up skin wounds, at first under close supervision. I started to get the hang of it. Applying exactly the right amount of tension in the loops of suture material was important. Making them too tight could cut off blood supply to the skin edges. Making them too loose could impede healing and produce wider scars. Spacing each suture correctly to close the wound neatly and achieving a secure and safe knot required discipline. I applied lessons learnt as a child from my carpenter father in his workshop, extending my index finger down the shaft of the needle-holder for maximum control. During my early clinical years, I had leaned towards being a physician, but I was learning to my surprise that I could be attracted to surgery.

9.

Steep Learning Curve

I CHOSE TO COMPLETE MY FINAL YEAR of study in Auckland. The idea of going to the country's most populous city to widen my experience made sense. My classmates and I had now gained the lofty status of 'trainee intern'. Along with this came greater responsibility. As well as attending formal lectures, we sometimes covered for absent house surgeons.

Although I had gained confidence and some basic skills in Tauranga, I was ill-prepared for emergencies. One night I was covering for a house surgeon in the ear, nose and throat surgical ward of Greenlane Hospital when I received a call. A few days earlier I had assisted in a routine adenoidectomy on a 20-year-old woman. Adenoids are small lumps of tissue at the back of the nose, above the roof of the mouth. When enlarged they can interfere with breathing. Their removal involves scraping around in the back of the throat with a sharp-edged spoon called a curette. This is accompanied by a nasty rasping sound as curette scrapes against bone, and by an alarming amount of bleeding. The operation had seemed barbaric.

Now the patient was having a major bleed. A bleed this long after an operation usually comes from an infection. I felt isolated and fearful. I had night nursing staff on hand but not an experienced doctor.

I sat the patient up, took blood for a crossmatch for a possible blood transfusion, put in an IV line and ran a saline drip full on.

I called for plasma. The bleeding continued unabated. The patient was becoming panic-stricken, her pulse rapid and her blood pressure dropping.

I knew this was an emergency: the patient could die. I quickly phoned my senior at his home. 'I have a patient with uncontrolled bleeding who is going flat,' I stammered out.

'I'll come in right away. Alert the operating theatre staff,' he said.

When he arrived after what seemed an age, he expertly packed the surgical area and stopped the bleeding. I was overcome with relief.

Steep Learning Curve

This emergency was a taste of more to come. Mostly I was loving this stimulating job, but there were certainly downsides.

Prizes were given in this final year for winning performances in clinical specialties, the plums being for medicine and surgery. I won a prize that I discovered was coveted by no one and ridiculed by some. It was for dermatology. The key to my success was my position on the senior Auckland University rugby team. The dermatologist who had examined us in a brief oral exam was a keen follower of the team. After a couple of easy questions, he'd asked me about the team's performance. This had led to an in-depth rugby discussion. We had got on well.

As January the first loomed, the day my classmates and I would show up for duty as fully qualified doctors, we jokingly warned friends and relatives to avoid entering a hospital that day. A batch of shiny new doctors, in our case the class of '68, would be let loose on an unsuspecting public.

At Auckland public hospitals, among which I was to rotate, the uniform was a crisp white full-length coat with voluminous pockets, in which we kept a stethoscope, a tendon hammer (to test reflexes), a safety pin, a tuning fork (to test sensation) and a notebook. We made a jangling sound as we swept around the ward. Attached to our belts or in our top pockets we sported a pager, always known as the bleeper.

Now began the years of assessing and admitting patients, then writing up their clinical notes; five and a half days a week of full-time work, with additional weeknights and weekends on call; interrupted sleep; scurrying around after seniors on ward rounds. Most junior doctors lived in accommodation in the hospital grounds, ready to be called on day and night. Pamela and I were no exception.

My first job on a 'run' (the term for duties with a particular team of consultants) involved general surgery, mainly abdominal. I liked the drama in theatre and the ability to fix things fast with direct hands-on action. My registrar, Harvey Morgan, was an enthusiastic teacher. He lived with his wife on a yacht moored in a marina close to the hospital, and one weekend took Pamela and me for a sail on Auckland harbour. The surgical run was a happy experience. Surgery was getting a tick on my preferred job list.

Next up was orthopaedics. The term 'orthopaedic' is derived from orthopédie, a term coined by an 83-year-old French doctor, Nicolas Andry de Bois-Regard, in 1741 from the Greek 'orthos', meaning correct or straight, and 'paidion', meaning child. The Tree of Andry – a crooked tree tied to an upright stake – has become the symbol for many orthopaedic organisations, including the New Zealand Orthopaedic Association.

Steep Learning Curve

Orthopaedics is concerned with disorders of the musculoskeletal system – muscles, bones and joints. Orthopaedic surgeons use both surgical and nonsurgical treatment methods. A large part of the job is treating patients with fractured bones, or dislocated joints that cause deformity or shortening of the limbs or spine. Correcting these involves a process called 'reduction'. Traction, pulling on the limb, overcomes the natural tendency of muscles to shorten the limb.

After the broken leg or arm or other bone has been straightened, it must be held in place until some healing takes place. This is done by encasing it in a plaster or fibreglass cast, or perhaps a removable splint. For severe fractures, a surgeon may need to operate, correcting the position of a limb and holding it with plates, screws, rods or wires. Since the 1960s, surgeons have also been replacing worn or diseased joints with artificial ones.

Sometimes, a surgeon or assistant has to put plenty of muscle into correcting injuries. Fixing a dislocated hip, for example, requires a major pull along the line of the femur. I once treated such a patient as he lay anaesthetised supine on the floor; I steadied his pelvis with my foot while I pulled the hip back into place. There was a satisfying 'thunk' as the ball of the femur returned to its home inside the hip socket. A similar technique with a foot in the armpit is sometimes used to correct a dislocated shoulder.

Blood and Bone

The orthopaedic ward was often dominated by young men with fractured femurs. Most had had motor vehicle accidents, commonly on a motorbike. We referred to them as sufferers of 'Kawasaki disease'– Kawasaki being a popular brand of motorbike. They were often noisy and boisterous, talking and joking loudly across cubicles with their fellow fracture-sufferers. Tied for months to their beds with traction weights strung over pulleys, they would become bored out of their minds. Visitors often brought them beer. The more enterprising enticed women to share their beds behind curtains during visiting hours. Any serious coupling would involve painful manoeuvres for the man and potentially also for the woman, who might get entangled in a rope or speared with a pin.

Middlemore Hospital was said to provide the largest orthopaedic service in the southern hemisphere. Being the only hospital in greater Auckland to accept acute cases, it was busy. As a junior house surgeon, the lowest rung on the ladder, I admitted patients downstairs then shot them up to my brother Garnet, who was by now working as an orthopaedic registrar. Garnet would manipulate, cast, apply traction or operate on those who needed it. If he had no cases to treat, he would come down and help me with admissions.

Garnet and I also combined on the rugby field. I had

again given up serious rugby for the backline of the medical boozers. Once, we played the navy at Devonport. They were a well-disciplined team of fit athletes; we were a ragtag team of sleep-deprived junior doctors.

Early in the game, ball in hand, I was going for the line with only one defender to beat. Next thing I remembered was halfway through the second half:

'What's the score?' I asked Garnet.

'I think you'd better go off the field,' he said.

From all accounts I had put out an arm to fend off the defender. A large man, he had grabbed my arm and propelled me with centrifugal force head-first into the ground. I'd got up a bit dazed and proceeded to tackle every naval thing that moved. Another of our team was taken to hospital injured. The navy didn't seem to do social.

I went back on call that night: there was nobody available to cover me at short notice. I reckoned I was anyway in an ideal place. If I had a bleed around the brain the other staff could quickly arrange for a burr hole to be made in my skull to drain the blood. Luckily none of this happened, but some colleagues said I should have had my head read.

A common injury we treated occurs in elderly women (and much less commonly in men) after a fall: hip fracture. After menopause, women's oestrogen levels drop, making their bones weaker, a condition called osteoporosis.

Hip fractures cause more hospitalisations among women than stroke, heart attack and breast cancer combined. Operating on patients with a fractured hip can get them mobile and increase their life expectancy.

Fracture of the neck of the femur requires surgery early to allow patients to walk. The operation fixes the head of the bone in its correct position. Nowadays a bone screw is used but in the '60s it was a threadless nail. The nail was driven across the fracture over a stout guide wire into the ball, then a side plate was attached to both the nail and the shaft of the femur below.

There was no X-ray machine to let us monitor the position of the guide wire as we inserted it. The operator simply pushed the wire where they thought it should be. A radiographer then wheeled a portable X-ray machine into the theatre and took a picture while the operating team trooped out, keeping our sterile gowns and gloved hands well clear of any unsterile object. When after several minutes the radiographer emerged from the darkroom, we peered at the image, pinned to a metal frame still dripping, and held up to the window. If the wire was not correctly positioned, the whole process was repeated.

One day my orthopaedic surgeon senior, Bill McFarland, made me an offer. If I could get the guide wire acceptably sited first try, three times in a row, on three separate patients, he would give me ten pounds. The wire had to be very close to the centre of the neck of the femur and the femoral head.

I took the bet. We both agreed the first two insertions were perfect. Then came the third. The key consideration: was the position 'acceptable'? A little leeway was allowable as long as the position would achieve a stable fix.

I held that my third effort was acceptable. I parroted the mantra he had taught me: 'The enemy of good is perfect.' This referred to the fact that sometimes, in siting metal implants in bone, adjusting a position from acceptable to ideal could end badly. The bone might crack, or a joint be entered by mistake. In this case the metal device was a fine-gauged wire, so if it was off-beam and entered the hip joint it would not cause a problem.

'Sorry,' Bill said. 'Not acceptable.' We trooped back in to adjust the position of the wire.

After six months I was deemed safe enough to cover the accident and emergency department, fondly known as A&E. There was no emergency medical specialty, so senior doctors were rarely available. Nobody at medical school had taught us how to treat many of the minor complaints and there was no internet to search. If a case was complex or a patient needed to be admitted, we would call the registrar of the appropriate specialty.

Some gave us a hard time if we cried for help too

readily. I learnt to trust the experienced nurses. 'What do I do now?' was a common request out of a patient's hearing.

Friday and Saturday nights were interesting as many patients were affected by alcohol. One drunk man was brought into A&E by his girlfriend in the early hours of the morning. He needed treatment for an injury sustained in a fight but was reluctant to let me examine him. I looked at his X-ray. He had a 'boxer's fracture'. This is a break at the neck of the little finger where the outside knuckle of the hand has been forced palm-wards. I asked the man how he'd injured his hand. 'Oh,' he said, 'I just put my hand out and the car door slammed into my palm.' I learnt from his partner that his fist had struck another man's jaw, an own goal.

I said to the plaster nurse, 'Let's cast this hand in a cobra back-slab.' This partial plaster-of-Paris cast is nicknamed 'cobra' because of its final shape – immobilised knuckle joints of the little finger and ring finger well bent, other finger joints bent a little, and wrist cocked backwards like a snake about to strike. The cast only partially encircles the injured part. Fully encircling an acutely injured finger or limb in a rigid cast risks the blood supply being cut off as the affected part swells inside the confined space.

I approached the patient. I overestimated his likely comprehension and cooperation. 'You've broken your hand at the little finger joint knuckle,' I explained. 'We will have to put it in plaster to ease your pain and allow your hand to heal in a satisfactory position. Your break isn't too bad. You will lose the prominence of the knuckle, but the hand should function normally after healing.'

There was silence. Then, 'I'm not having no plaster and you can fuck off.' He was almost paralytic. His girlfriend restrained him while I gave him the snake.

Severe hand injuries are treated by both plastic and orthopaedic surgeons in New Zealand. At Middlemore we worked closely with the plastic surgery department, which dealt with the most complex cases. I appreciated the clear explanations of the basic principles for treating these injuries by Joan Chapple, a plastic and hand surgeon and a charismatic teacher. The key requirement was for the patient to end up with a fully flexible hand. 'It's all very well to end up with a healed fracture, but if the hand is stiff the patient won't thank you.'

Joan discouraged us from using immobilising splinting for fractured fingers. Where the bone fragments are mostly in line or only a little displaced, the finger will heal well, even with a little movement. She favoured 'buddy-strapping' – using the finger next to the injured one as the splint and encouraging the patient to move both fingers. Her words are still clear in my mind 50 years later. I often take off rigid splints put on by doctors who've treated a patient before me. I was to discover that booze-sodden A&E customers are not a uniquely New Zealand phenomenon. Two years later I was the recipient of alcohol-induced violence while working at Plymouth Hospital in Devon, England. A child with a broken arm was brought in by his father, who was clearly intoxicated. I decided to treat the fracture under general anaesthetic. The boy had just eaten. I said to his father, 'I'm afraid we won't be able to put your son to sleep for about four hours. There is a danger that, with his full stomach, he may inhale its contents, which is dangerous.'

The father stood up. He was in an angry mood. I remonstrated. 'Please sit down.' Bad move: I found myself on the ground with broken spectacles. Luckily, the police station was next to the hospital and the man was swiftly removed. From then on I treated drunks with greater caution. I learnt the technique of swallowing rats and biting my tongue. I addressed them as 'sir', spoke with nauseating sweetness and trod carefully.

Despite some anxious times and mistakes made, I enjoyed A&E. I triaged patients and treated those I could. I cleaned, anaesthetised and sutured skin wounds; helped manipulate and plaster simple fractures and fixed simple joint dislocations; and pumped out drugs from the stomachs of suicidal patients – almost always young females and often non-lethal doses. I assessed serious head and other injuries from car accidents, started the emergency procedures, ordered X-rays and tests and called seniors for help. I would quickly discharge patients with minor conditions and admit others. I enjoyed the quick-fire nature of the work: solve one problem, then on to the next.

Removing foreign bodies from patients was a common task. Extracting broken needles from feet was tricky. An X-ray would guide me as to where to make an incision in the locally anaesthetised skin, but sometimes I couldn't find the needle. The fat pad of the heel is like the proverbial haystack, except that haystacks don't bleed. I learnt that if I couldn't find the needle fairly quickly after fossicking around, I should ring the orthopaedic registrar. He or she would sometimes have to admit the patient and, while they were under general anaesthetic, apply a thigh tourniquet to create a near bloodless field.

One of the more interesting items I had to remove was a stingray spine. The young man had been starting out for a bit of fun in the surf. 'I ran from the beach into the water and felt a sudden severe pain,' he told me. 'I kicked but the stingray lost and I gained.' Stingray spines are sharp and can be toxic. It took a while to carefully remove it.

Later, as a registrar, I removed another foreign body notorious for breeding infection: a phoenix palm frond. These injuries are surprisingly common. According to ACC, there were 741 claims for phoenix palm injuries in New Zealand in 2019.

When these sharp fronds puncture the skin, usually feet or hands, they cause a lot of pain. In this case, the frond had lodged in a young woman's foot for several days before she showed up at A&E. By then most of her foot was inflamed. After I operated to remove the frond and clean out the infection, she spent several days in hospital with her foot elevated, receiving industrial doses of intravenous antibiotics.

I heard from colleagues and read that all sorts of foreign bodies end up in places where the sun doesn't shine. The rectum and vagina are a temporary home for a variety of objects: candles (popular), dildos, coins, children's toys, bottles, jewellery. The urethra has been used to accommodate metallic cables, plastic tubes, fish, and in one recorded case a snake. It was not recorded whether the snake was retrieved dead or alive.

I often felt inadequate. One night a patient presented after a fight. His ear was lacerated and held on to his skull by a sliver of skin. With his stubbly beard he bore an uncanny resemblance to Vincent van Gogh. I had that anxious out-of-my-depth feeling. I rang the plastic surgeon on call and still remember his exact words: 'Catgut to the subcutaneous and mersilk to the skin and you can do it.' He didn't know me from Adam. I think his faith in me was largely due to the lateness of the night and his discomfort at the prospect of coming to the hospital.

I was proud of the result: the ear firmly stayed on after I'd finished and looked similar, if not in exactly the same position, to the man's other ear.

However, one of my mistakes caused a tragedy. In the early hours of the morning, a Polynesian couple brought in their baby. The child was feverish and breathing rapidly, with an alarming wheeze. I diagnosed bronchiolitis, a common viral infection in babies and young children that causes inflammation and congestion in the small airways of the lung. Most children get better with care at home. A small percentage require hospitalisation.

I rang the paediatrician on call at Princess Mary Hospital for Children, 17 kilometres away. 'Excuse me, doctor,' I said, 'I have a three-month-old child with bronchiolitis – pallid colour with a very rapid respiratory rate and major wheeze. We're giving the child humidified oxygen with a little improvement. Should I send him over to you?'

The doctor sounded sleepy. He suggested keeping the baby a bit longer. When his breathing settled I should discharge him for 'more definitive treatment' the next day if he hadn't improved. I felt uncomfortable but was not confident enough to insist on the baby being admitted. About three hours later he returned, dead in his mother's arms. I was devastated. I had learnt an important lesson: I had to trust my instincts and be more assertive.

My next run made me reject a career as a physician – a specialist in general or internal medicine known in the

United States as an internist. 'Internal' was originally used to describe this kind of medicine to differentiate it from 'external' medicine – surgery. Today physicians diagnose and treat a wide variety of conditions, often complex, with an emphasis on prescribing medicines.

My new bosses were good to work with and I liked their meticulous and considered approach, but the work didn't suit me. It was too slow. By the end of three or four hours trudging around the ward as the junior member of the retinue, I was bored. The specialists seemed compelled to listen to almost every patient's chest, even when lungs and heart didn't seem to be the problem. Tiny adjustments were made to medication on a 'let's see what happens' basis. There seemed little sense of urgency. Patients stayed for days or weeks in the ward.

At the end of my first ward round with the physicians there was an unpleasant surprise. We filed into the sluice room. There, lined up and carefully named, were the recent contents of the large bowel of several of our patients. One of the consultants was a gastroenterologist. We had not been told as students that diagnosis in this specialty required close observation of faeces. I had learnt to breathe through my mouth when confronted with bad patient smells, but this was a new level. Come the end of the ward round, not only was I tired and bored but I had a very dry mouth.

Steep Learning Curve

I was finding I liked quick results. The A&E run had been all action – meet, treat, relieve pain, correct any abnormality, discharge the patient or refer them on. On general surgery, the ward rounds had been smart and focused: prepare patients for surgery and care for them afterwards. The medical run, by comparison, lacked drama – except when there was a cardiac arrest, which seemed to occur mostly in the middle of the night. Then there was too much drama.

My next run was paediatrics. I was looking at this as a possible specialty, but I often found the work disturbing, especially cannulating veins and administering intravenous chemotherapy to child cancer victims. Having to hurt these acutely unwell children was hard. I hated causing them pain.

I was almost unable to deal with my own pain during one unfortunate episode. I received a call from a nurse: 'Can you go to room number three – the kid with the massive hydrocephalus has just burst his head.' I'd never heard of such an awful event. I quickly went to the child. Sure enough, his huge skull, grossly swollen because of a blockage to the drainage system of cerebrospinal fluid in the brain, had eventually given way. His forehead was flat. Fluid soaked the pillow. I could hardly look.

He was still breathing. What on earth should I do? I rang my registrar. 'Get a large dose of morphine and give it intravenously,' he said. 'We don't want the child to suffer.'

I extinguished the child's life. I was a mess.

Part of my discomfort treating children was probably due to my own early experiences. As a child I had a terror of needles. One time our mother told us our family doctor was coming to inject us – I think it must have been for a vaccination. Back then GPs visited patients at home for routine treatments. From my hiding place behind a pile of bricks at the back door, I heard my mother's anxious voice. 'Russy, where are you? The doctor's here. Come on.' I bent lower. I wasn't going anywhere near the needle-wielding doctor.

'Russell, come here at once!' My mother sounded cross. Soon, I heard the doctor slam his car door and drive off. I was safe.

Nowadays there are ways of lessening the pain, and therefore the fear, that children feel when medical professionals must perform potentially painful procedures on them. Topical local anaesthetic preparations numb skin prior to needles being inserted. Our little patients had no such luck. We forcibly restrained them while trying to insert drips, a life-saving procedure for dehydrated children with high fevers. These were exacting technical exercises: tiny veins were sometimes difficult to enter, even with the finest of needles.

We admitted many feverish babies. The instinct of some mothers was to wrap these sick children in layers

Steep Learning Curve

of clothing. Unfortunately, this raised their body temperature even higher. As a result, some had febrile convulsions, disturbing to witness. I was taught that the correct initial treatment for a very hot child was to strip off their clothes and, if necessary, cool them by partial immersion in cold water until their body temperature dropped, at the same time keeping their head dry. This is still the same today.

As a house surgeon, being on call at nights and weekends was exhausting. On one three-month rotation, I covered a general medical ward on a one-in-two roster. Every second night and weekend I would work a normal day and then be available for work that night, finishing at the end of the next day. This meant, for the weekdays, a minimum of about 33 hours either at work or on call. After a normal day's work and one night off, it started all over again.

I managed to get home before falling asleep in front of patients but a few times, having collapsed into bed, I was called back to the hospital to resuscitate a patient suffering cardiac arrest or another medical emergency. At such times I functioned well under par. So did my conscientious registrar. On one occasion in the early morning hours he fell asleep and had to be woken up by the patient he was examining.

After this run I was scheduled to join the critical care team. The head was a doctor known to be highly dedicated but gruff and demanding. Some juniors loved the drama of treating the sickest patients in the hospital and the senior staff supported them well. But with my one-in-two call roster fresh in my mind, I phoned him. 'Doctor, I'm scheduled to work with you on my next rotation, which I'm looking forward to. But I recently worked a one-in-two and found it very exhausting. Would it be possible to work a one-in-three roster with you?'

'No,' he replied. 'You'll never be able to keep up with your patients on that schedule. I will not have doctors on my run who won't fit into our routines.'

I thanked him and rang off. I did geriatrics instead.

10.

The Locum Life

WHEN I'D FIRST OBSERVED SURGERY, I'd felt an aversion. But as a house surgeon I'd found I loved it – the challenge of mastering the techniques, the discipline, the close teamwork, and particularly the atmosphere in the operating theatre. I liked the need for quick decision-making and gained satisfaction from seeing a patient quickly restored to health.

Having decided on a surgical career, the first hurdle I faced was part one of the surgical fellowship. A senior colleague persuaded me I should go to the UK to do it through the Royal College of Surgeons. This had appeal. The pass rate for New Zealanders was usually significantly higher than for the corresponding New Zealand exam. Also, most candidates for the New Zealand exam spent a year in Dunedin working and studying at the medical school. I thought five years there had been enough.

Most of my fellow junior doctors were going to spend two years as house surgeons but I decided on 18 months. That way I could travel to London in time for the four-month course at Nuffield College, which began towards the end of the year. Pamela and I could then do the traditional OE before coming home.

Some of my Auckland colleagues issued dire warnings. Having left New Zealand on this 'jaunt' (as they saw it), I would, they said, have trouble getting a job back home later. I saw no evidence for this and went ahead with my plans. I first needed time to study for the entry exam. Luckily, the geriatrics run at Cornwall Hospital was not too taxing, I liked working with the elderly patients. Their conditions were mainly chronic and treatment was spare. The light workload gave me ample time to study and I passed the exam well.

The next question was how to afford life in London. Although Pamela was working full-time as a secondary school teacher, we were not making enough to pay the fees for my full-time course at the Royal College of Surgeons, let alone save for accommodation and living expenses. I decided to take a job as a locum in Ponsonby.

The Locum Life

It's July 1970, early on a winter's morning in Auckland's inner-city suburb. The phone rings by my bed. I wake disoriented. I've not long gone to sleep after a 13-hour day's work during an influenza outbreak. The GP I'm covering is on holiday. I've never done a locum before.

'Doctor, my father's not feeling well. He's been a bit crook all evening but now he's taken a turn for the worse. He's complaining of chest pain.'

The caller tells me her father is 68 and has no history of chest or heart problems. 'He's a good colour and not too bad, but I'm a bit worried. He normally keeps well and doesn't complain when he's not.'

I question her about the chest pain. Does it go up into his neck or down his arm? 'I think it's a bit sharp when he breathes in,' she says.

She yells to her father. 'Dad, does it go into your neck or arm?'

'He says no,' she reports.

I ask for more details. Does he feel hot? Might he have a temperature?

'I think he might,' she says, 'but I don't have a thermometer.'

I'm reluctant to get out of bed. I'm desperately tired. I know I have another full day's work ahead, with about 30 patients to see in the clinic and maybe some home visits.

I ask a few more questions. In retrospect they were

leading questions, rather than open ones that avoid putting ideas and words into the mouths of patients or their relatives. I'm thinking the caller's father most likely has the flu, like many patients I've seen the day before. The sharp nature of the pain when he breathes in may mean he has pleurisy, an infection involving the lining of the lung. I assure myself that I needn't visit him immediately.

'Cool his forehead and skin with a moist flannel, give him two paracetamol tablets and get him to drink plenty of water. I'll come round first thing in the morning but do ring me if he gets worse.'

I fall back to sleep.

Half an hour later, the phone rings again. 'Doctor, can you come round. Dad's got worse chest pain. It's there all the time now, getting more severe and he says it's heavy and he's finding it hard to breathe.'

I ask her to ring for an ambulance and say it's urgent, then I quickly dress and rush out the door. I drive quickly. By the time I get to the house the man is unconscious. I feel for his pulse. There isn't one.

'Quick, help me get him onto the floor,' I say to the daughter. I start resuscitation, compressing the man's chest rhythmically and breathing for him, mouth to mouth. Twenty minutes later, I give up.

The ambulance arrives but it's too late. I've failed this man and his family. I'm distraught. I had misdiagnosed the symptoms during the first phone call, fervently hoping it wasn't heart pain. The pain of a heart attack is not usually sharp, but it can be. I should have gone around to the house immediately to assess him myself, not relied on second-hand information. The failure to do this still haunts me.

I was ill-equipped to cope with the role of a busy general practitioner. My experience and training for general practice had been minimal. As a medical student I had a few times sat alongside a GP in his clinic, merely looking on. Since graduating I had worked for 18 months as a house surgeon, but under the supervision of senior doctors.

A more experienced doctor would have handled the workload better. Established GPs get to know their patients and can assess their health needs better than a locum treating a patient completely unknown to them. Today no rookie doctor would do this work without supervision. I was green and over-confident – I didn't know what I didn't know.

The next challenge was how to get to London. Air travel was beyond our means. I took on a job as doctor on a Shaw Saville merchant navy ship. The deal for the five-week journey was a free trip for me and $90 for Pamela's expenses. We were glad we didn't have to pay for the meals. There was no fresh food from New Zealand; we dined on what remained from the ship's voyage from the UK. The kippers served up for breakfast smelled strongly and tasted the same. Pamela was in the early stages of pregnancy and couldn't stomach them, or much else. Our daughter, born in Plymouth after we arrived, appeared to have suffered no ill effects from Pamela's diet of boiled eggs.

Doctors were an unusual luxury on Shaw Saville ships, hired only when hospitalised or disabled sailors had to be returned home after being treated in New Zealand. Before the ship left, I inspected the medical equipment and drugs on board. The cupboard was virtually bare. There was a large bottle of black sticky liquid, with instructions for the dose needed for a wide variety of medical conditions. This went something like 'one teaspoon three times a day for piles, two teaspoons for an itchy rash, three teaspoons for heartburn'. I wondered whether some hapless sailor might have been prescribed half a bottle for acute appendicitis. (There was no instruction for this condition.) There was no local anaesthetic. Any lacerations were apparently sown up without it.

I stocked up on medicines, including a generous supply of long-acting penicillin. As it turned out my daily clinics were often empty and I didn't use most of the medicines, suturing only a few small wounds (under local anaesthetic) and tending other minor complaints. But the penicillin was a hit. The sailors told me they'd had a good

The Locum Life

time in port at Durban and Cape Town so I prescribed it lavishly following our stops there. The black medicine remained unused.

The Royal College of Surgeons of England (RCSE) is descended from the Barber-Surgeons' Company, established in 1540 by an act of parliament in the reign of Henry VIII. Divorced from the barbers in 1745, the Company of Surgeons eventually became The Royal College of Surgeons of London, and in 1843 the RCSE. The Nuffield College of Surgical Sciences, where I studied, was housed in an austere building in Lincoln's Inn Field, a large public square. Originally it had been located close to Newgate Prison, a handy source of bodies for dissection.

The course just before mine had been the last at Nuffield for Professor Raymond Last, reputed to be a superb anatomy teacher. Last had been a practising surgeon in Adelaide, Australia before becoming an anatomist. His textbook *Last's Anatomy: Regional and Applied*, which we used, was clinically oriented. I was particularly fascinated by Last's description of the anatomy of the knee, which taught me much I had not learned at medical school.

I was disappointed that Last was no longer teaching, but Frank Stansfield, who took his place, turned out to be one of the best teachers I ever had. His sense of humour was famous. His entry in *Plarr's Lives of the Fellows*, a collection of biographies, notes that his 'imparting of his encyclopaedic knowledge of anatomy was accompanied by quirkish witticisms provoked by faltering and erroneous answers to questions, e.g. "That is positively grotesque. You are anticipating backwards and retrospecting the future. We go at one speed and one speed only: dead slow".'

'What is a lecture?' he would say. 'It is words proceeding from the mouth of the speaker to the notebooks of his pupils without entering the brains of either.'

And: 'What is revision? It is learning something for the first time one week before the examination.'

I fondly remember one of his drole one-liners. 'What is the function of the tonsil?' he asked. Someone in the class mumbled the correct answer. 'No,' he said, 'it is to provide the means, when removed, to allow the ENT surgeon to acquire his next brand-new Rolls Royce.'

As I prepared to sit the primary exam I remembered a tip a colleague who had been through the course had given me. 'Swot up hydatids thoroughly, then make sure you wear an Otago Medical School tie to the viva [the oral part of the exam].'

Hydatids, eradicated in New Zealand since 2002, was then a fairly common disease. Its tapeworms were carried by sheep and other livestock. Dogs eating the offal of infected sheep got tapeworms in their intestines. Humans became infected by eating food contaminated by dog faeces that contained tapeworm eggs. The eggs became larvae, which burrowed through the human intestine to lodge in one of many internal organs, most commonly the liver. There, large cysts containing many small tapeworms caused abdominal pain or, if the cyst ruptured, death.

'Good morning, Dr Tregonning,' the examiner said. 'Please sit down.' After a few short questions he said, 'I see you have a medical tie on. Where is it from? Ah, from New Zealand? You will no doubt know something about hydatid disease then. Please tell me about the cause, pathology and symptoms of hydatid disease of the liver.'

I could hardly believe my luck. I regurgitated the textbook description in full detail. The bell sounded. End of viva.

Of the four New Zealanders at the college, three of us passed. We partied long and hard that night. The only downer was thinking about our friend who had failed; we had to drink a bit more to drown our sorrows on his behalf. (He would subsequently pass the exam and become a fine surgeon.)

After gaining the first part of the surgical fellowship, I travelled extensively with Pamela through Europe, England and Ireland. We had bought a second-hand dormobile, naïvely trusting the New Zealander who sold it to us.

On a trial run around southern England, I drove too close to a truck and broke off a side mirror. It was a portent. The man who'd sold us the dormobile had failed to carry out the agreed-upon repairs. Not far from Rome an internal pipe blew up. Pamela, in the passenger seat, had to try and plug the flow of hot radiator water with a towel.

To keep travelling we needed to top up our funds. I answered an advertisement for a locum in downtown Edinburgh. When I went for an interview, the GP was not present. I gathered he was elderly. The practice nurse showed me the small office. The examination room was dark and musty, the couch piled high with issues of *British Medical Journal*. 'I see the couch is out of commission,' I said. 'Where does Dr McPherson examine his patients if he needs them to lie down?'

'Och, if they need that sort of examination he sends them up to the Infirmary,' she replied, referring to the Edinburgh Royal Infirmary.

When I took the job, I cleared a space on the couch. I wanted to know what was wrong with my patients' abdomens, backs, hips or knees if I was to consider referring them to the infirmary.

My next locum was covering Edinburgh's Portobello and Craigentinny suburbs. I found my patients charming. I loved hearing their accents and quaint expressions and realised it was much the way my mother's Scottish father

The Locum Life

would have spoken. On one home visit the patient was an elderly retired man who'd had a minor fall. We started to chat. His brother had migrated to New Zealand, he said. I told him of my Scottish blood. 'Would ye care for a wee dram, doctor?' he inquired. I did care and was warmed by a shot of whisky.

Back in England we needed to put down roots as Pamela was now heavily pregnant. I was keen to explore my ancestry in Cornwall but couldn't find a hospital job in the capital, Truro. I accepted a job as senior house officer in A&E at Plymouth Hospital just across the border in Devon.

I was fascinated to hear the accent that my Tregonning great-grandparents would have had and the common expression 'Allo, moi luverr' ('Hello, my lover'). At work I wore walk shorts and long socks, the standard Auckland hospital uniform for juniors. I was a curiosity. Locals whistled at me as I walked through the town.

One morning I woke to find Pamela in pain. Although she was nine months pregnant, I was sure it wasn't labour. I diagnosed a bladder problem, and reassured by my diagnostic skills went off to work. About an hour later I was called to the phone. It was Pamela. 'Come quickly, I'm having the baby.' I raced home, got her into the dormobile and sped to the maternity ward. I was allowed into the delivery room but firmly told I'd have to leave if there were problems with the birth. There were, but in their haste to deliver the distressed baby with forceps the midwives forgot about me.

I was embarrassed about my initial misdiagnosis. In my defence, the baby's head had presented the wrong way round. This had caused pressure on Pamela's bladder, which accounted for her continuous low abdominal pain. Perhaps if I'd completed the prescribed number of deliveries before graduation I'd have learnt this lesson?

The baby was a girl. We called her Camilla. She was the most beautiful creature I had ever seen. As I pushed her through the town in her pram, my heart bursting with pride, I wore long trousers.

11.

Final Judgement

AFTER 14 MONTHS AWAY, WE RETURNED to New Zealand. It was time for the next stage of surgical training. I was accepted into the Auckland Hospitals' scheme. I would work as a registrar before sitting the final exam to become a fully qualified surgeon. Once more, though, a top-up of funds was required. I took on a locum for a country GP in Owaka, a small town in Otago, close to south-east tip of the South Island. My maternal roots were at nearby Kaitangata: my Scottish grandfather had been a coal miner there, my grandmother a part-time musician and mother of eight.

The practice covered the large and sparsely populated

Catlins, a rugged and beautiful part of New Zealand I came to love. I had the use of my employer's car, a grunty Triumph that nearly did me in. I'd never driven such a powerful car. The roads outside Owaka were unsealed. One day on a trip back from a clinic at Tokanui, a town 75 kilometres away, I got into a skid taking a heavily gravelled corner too fast. The car soared off the road. Fortunately, it and I remained upright.

Another nasty experience was being called to Kaka Point for an emergency in the dead of night. I was travelling by memory from directions I'd been given over the phone. I had no knowledge of the geography, no useful map, and in 1971 no mobile phone, GPS or satnav. Lost and panicking, I somehow finally happened upon the right place. By then I was more in need of treatment than the patient.

In 1972 we bought a house in Māngere in South Auckland with a large mortgage and I started the first of four six-monthly rotations – three in general surgery and one in orthopaedics. In general surgery, we treated many patients with conditions that are very common in New Zealand: breast cancer and bowel cancer. For some advanced breast cancers we undertook radical mastectomies, which involved removing not only the breast but also the underlying chest muscles, even if there was no cancer there. This was common in the early 1970s.

Final Judgement

I did not like assisting with this disfiguring operation. Today, it is rarely performed as surgery for breast cancer has become much less invasive. Lumpectomy – removal of the lump alone – combined with radiation therapy is now acceptable treatment for some cancers.

Operating for cancer of the large bowel meant cutting out the tumour and then sewing together the cut ends of the bowel. The cancer is sometimes deep in the pelvis, close to the junction of the colon and rectum. I found the surgery difficult, with the ever-present threat of a dangerous leakage at the join afterwards. I struggled to master the technique. I was learning that general surgery wasn't for me.

One of my fellow surgical trainees, Richard, had the nickname 'chopper'. When he was a Dunedin medical student, his hostel mates reported that when someone had locked him out of his room he took the quick way in, cutting through the door with an axe. Richard would go on to become head of paediatric heart units in Australia and the United States, where his work involved highly skilled and fine manipulation of new-born children's hearts the size of walnuts. He became internationally known, lectured and demonstrated in operating theatres across the world, and developed a new operation for a lethal condition in which a baby is born with the two largest arteries in the body placed the wrong way around.

Early on, Richard demonstrated his sewing skills. We met up in Wanaka on holiday and camped overnight up the Wilkin River flats. At dawn we shot a deer. I was the assistant and Richard the surgeon as we dismembered the animal for meat to take home. Suddenly, Richard's hunting knife slipped. I reeled back, clutching a wound bleeding freely just above my eyebrow.

Firm binding with a pillow slip around my head stemmed the flow as we continued our work, then packed out our gear and meat and went to stay with his wife's parents nearby. Fortunately, Richard had brought suture material and local anaesthetic. His father-in-law, a farmer, calmly hoed into bacon and eggs as Richard sewed me up at the other end of the kitchen table. I can attest to his skill: the scar is barely visible.

When we occasionally operated in tandem at Auckland Hospital, Richard's sureness and dexterity were obvious. During one operation, the removal of a diseased gall bladder, I was blown away by his speed and skill. I felt a complete klutz and worried that I was in the wrong job. I ignored this disturbing idea: I had come too far to turn back.

The orthopaedic run, by contrast with general surgery, was all cool instruments and shiny hardware and I found the techniques relatively simple. The operative field was clean – no nasty bowel contents – and disfiguring removal of normal tissue was usually not needed. The exception was limb amputations, but they were becoming less and less common as reconstructive surgery for mangled limbs and unusual musculoskeletal cancers improved. The people I worked with were quite relaxed and the manual skills echoed those I'd used in my dad's workshop. I felt at home.

The two orthopaedic chiefs on my first run were particularly easy-going. Both smoked heavily. On ward rounds, if they were still smoking as we approached the patients' six-bedded cubicle, each would leave his glowing cigarette on the ledge outside. Then it was a quick pick-up-and-drag on the way out before facing the patients in the next cubicle.

One of these men was a keen fly-fisherman. When he'd received his surgical fellowship, he'd hung up his stethoscope in his office. He reasoned that as an orthopaedic surgeon he wouldn't be listening to hearts, lungs or abdomens ever again. Whenever he wore out the feathers on his dry flies, he would hook them into the red rubber tubing of the stethoscope.

He was a character, great to work with, helpful and never judgemental. He had started life as a carpenter and had no airs or graces. He used to regale us at morning tea with his exploits on the rugby field. Having played in the front row of the scrum, he revealed some of the dark arts practised far from the referee's watchful eye. Later, he gave up smoking and chewed prodigious amounts of chewing gum in theatre. I can still see his mask moving up and down as he rhythmically crushed the great wad of gum behind it.

The demands of my job placed stresses on family life. Trying to balance the opposing demands on my time and energy led to difficulties with a small number of senior colleagues. These men (none were women) were accomplished doctors, hard-working and dedicated to their patients, but their expectations of young doctors took little account of changing times and the increasing focus on work-life balance.

There was no union. Any negotiations with hospital employers were dependent on voluntary action by groups of junior doctors, meeting after hours. We had little time or energy for vigorous industrial activity, even if we thought it appropriate. And not everyone did.

We were dependent on our medical bosses for promotion. Some of them were not happy with any request to improve our working conditions. Their main argument seemed to be: we had conditions the same as yours, or even worse. What are you on about? There was no mention of the fact that if we didn't cover them day and night, they might have to come in after hours to treat acutely injured patients.

Later, one of my bosses, the departmental head at Wellington Hospital, was on call with me one weekend.

Final Judgement

He took me aside. 'Russell,' he said, 'I'm going up the coast. I don't expect to be called.' Although I was flattered by his confidence in me, I was still officially under his supervision. In the event of a multiple trauma situation with a bad car crash or a similar accident, I was supposed to call him. His attitude seemed to me a dereliction of his duty to his patients: it was his name on the board at the end of every bed.

In the middle of 1973 Pamela was admitted to National Women's Hospital after I had, this time, successfully diagnosed labour. Once there I made a blue. After several hours Pamela was crying out for something to cool her dry mouth. Knowing her weakness for ice cream and chocolate, I returned to her bedside with two large chocolate bombs. We were munching contentedly when the midwife arrived. 'Dr Tregonning,' she said, 'what on earth do you think you're doing? You should know better. Your wife may need a general anaesthetic – you're endangering her.' Fortunately, my brain fade caused no harm. Pamela did not need a general anaesthetic. An uncomplicated delivery produced our son Mark.

Four months later it was time for me to sit the big one – the final examination of the Royal Australasian College of Surgeons. Remarkably, among others there was another question on hydatids. I dredged up all I knew and wrote a brilliant (in my opinion) answer. I owe a lot to this disease, even though I helped with operations for it only two or three times when I was on surgical runs.

Then came the oral exam. I was amazed how nervous I was. The examiner was a general surgeon with a reputation for terrorising candidates. I was outwardly calm, but a seething mess inside.

'Dr Tregonning, please describe how you would perform an emergency tracheotomy on a child.' I had never been involved in such an operation, let alone on a child. I'd read about it, but that was a long time ago.

I flailed around. I imagined myself failing and having to re-sit this important exam months later. By good fortune I'd never failed an important exam but now my time had come. My incompetence was obvious.

To buy time, I long-windedly began describing the positioning of the patient and skin preparation. 'We'll take that as read, doctor. Describe your incision and the next steps.'

I described the incision of the trachea.

'What scalpel blade will you use?'

I hadn't learnt this. In fact, I'd done almost no paediatric surgery. I blurted out, 'That long sharp pointy one.'

My answer was so ridiculous the examiner smiled, clearly amused by my ineptitude. 'You mean the number eleven blade, don't you?'

Final Judgement

I quickly recovered. 'Oh yes, of course.'

My ignorance of the number eleven blade could have spelt a fail. Ironically, it would become my favourite blade. During my career I would use it more often than any other, making the skin portals for keyhole surgery on knees. I rejoice in the number eleven blade.

Somehow I passed. At the function afterwards, we were supposed to drink sherry with our examiners, a tradition. The sherry had run out. We drank something stronger. There was a god after all.

A less serious complication was to come. My patient was Grant Nisbett, the well-known rugby commentator, affectionately known New Zealand-wide as 'Nisbo'. A day after I had performed his knee replacement, the head operating theatre nurse called me. 'Russell, can you come over to view Mr. Nisbett's knee X-ray.' I felt immediate anxiety. I was never called to be told what a good job I'd done. Sure enough, there was a fine guide rod in the left femur inserted to help align the prosthesis precisely. It should have been removed. While I had flexed the knee, the wire had been pushed inside the bone where I couldn't see it. The instrument tray had only one slot for two such guide wires. The scrub nurse saw one correctly in place and didn't recognise the other was missing. As is always our routine, she told me that all the instruments were removed, thus giving me permission to close the wound.

I immediately apologised to Grant. I told him that it would not likely cause any trouble as we routinely leave large thick metal rods in femurs after fracture fixation. Check X-rays showed no rod migration.

Just before Grant left hospital, I made a suggestion, 'Grant, can we cut a deal? If you don't tell the nation about this episode, we'll name the rod after you – "the Nisbo".' He was generous and agreed. From then on, before wound closure, I called out, 'have we removed the Nisbo?' By then I had changed my technique. We always had.

12.

Joining the Herd

AMONG THE (MOSTLY) GOOD-NATURED insults hurled at orthopaedic surgeons by other doctors is that we are 'strong as oxen and twice as bright'. Adam Kay, author of the bestseller *This is Going to Hurt: Secret Diaries of a Junior Doctor*, describes orthopaedics as 'basically reserved for the med school's rugby team – it's barely more than sawing and nailing – and I suspect they don't "sign up" for it so much as dip their hand in ink and provide a palm print.'

Kay, an obstetrician and gynaecologist who gave up medicine to become a fulltime writer and comedian, is right to some extent: 'sawing' is still a big part of modern joint replacement surgery. Although amputations have become unusual, modern surgeons regularly saw off worn-out or diseased joint surfaces, replacing them with prosthetic components. But 'barely more than sawing and nailing' implies that orthopaedic surgeons don't need much skill. Not so. Hand surgery requires a delicate touch and gentle handling of tissue. Spinal surgeons dice with permanent and disastrous neurological injury. Knee surgery and keyhole surgery – arthroscopy – use delicate instruments that require fine motor skills.

The FRACS examination was a generic surgical qualification. My further training in orthopaedics was to take four more years. The Auckland hospital orthopaedic teams consisted mainly of part-time consultants visiting from their private practices. After I was chosen for the training, I was approached by the powerbroker of Auckland orthopaedics, whom I just thought of as 'the boss'. He invited me to work with him for six months. I was flattered. In the 1960s he had set up a scoliosis unit to correct spinal deformity at Middlemore Hospital and the Ōtara spinal unit for spinal injuries (now called the Auckland Spinal Rehabilitation Unit). He had helped develop hip replacement surgery at Middlemore Hospital, the orthopaedic academic unit at the University of Auckland and the NZOA registrar training programme. In the 1996 book *Orthopaedics in New Zealand*, fellow orthopaedic surgeon Colin Hooker would describe him as 'An outstanding figure in New Zealand orthopaedics … he has probably contributed as much as any other person to the advancement of the specialty in New Zealand and to bring New Zealand orthopaedic surgery onto the world scene.'

But as time went on the boss would create major problems for me. To gain an overseas job, younger surgeons often depended on patronage from seniors. The boss helped me gain a post in Toronto. I would take this up in 1976. Meanwhile, there was a quid pro quo: my career was at least partially under his control. My weekday roster of one-in-five sounded relatively benign. The catch was that the boss's on-call weekday was Friday, the busiest night of the week. The weekend 'on call' for me therefore ran from eight on Friday morning to Monday morning, followed by a full day's normal work. Potentially, it was 80 hours of work. The orthopaedic acute service at Middlemore Hospital covered the greater Auckland area, population then about 750,000. Each weekend on call would bring acute trauma cases up to high double figures both days. There was no break. I sometimes barely slept for three nights.

After one such weekend I entered the lion's den. I said, 'I wonder if the roster can be altered to change your weeknight on call from Friday. I'm finding the four-night weekend gruelling, and I fear my ability to treat patients may be affected when I'm so tired.'

'No, Russell, that won't be happening,' he said. 'I've always had this arrangement.'

I later heard from one of his senior colleagues that he liked Friday on call as the large number of cases meant his patients were spread around the other wards after his own was full. His name, therefore, appeared on the board at every nurse's station and at end of many beds. My junior colleagues and I were less than impressed by this. Run off our feet from the weekend's work, we had to trudge far and wide to service patients in these other wards in the days and weeks afterwards.

I worked closely with three younger consultants who were full-time at the hospitals: Brian Otto and Bill Gillespie at Middlemore Hospital and John Cullen at Auckland Hospital. Bill was to have a particularly strong influence on my career. A graduate of Edinburgh, he was on a year-long exchange in Auckland. Later, he became professor of orthopaedics successively at Christchurch, Newcastle in Australia and Edinburgh. He went on to become dean of the Otago Medical School and finally foundation dean of the Hull York Medical School in the UK when it opened in 2003. Bill's stellar career was marked by his encouraging doctors to develop teaching and research roles alongside their clinical duties. On a personal level, I was grateful to him for relieving me on Sundays when I desperately needed sleep after continuous four-day work marathons at Middlemore.

When admitting a patient, we went through the time-honoured routines, the basic foundations of clinical diagnosis that had been drilled into us. We took and recorded their 'history' – their account of their current injury or disease – and asked about the medicines they were taking. We asked about their previous illnesses and allergies (the 'past' history) and about their living conditions and family illnesses (the 'social' and 'family' histories). We examined them, looking carefully and feeling their bodies for areas of tenderness or deformity. We assessed the range of motion of their joints – both 'passive' (where we helped move the joint) and 'active' (where the patient moved their joint to the max). All these were encapsulated in the mantra *Look, Feel, Move*, which I had been taught and would later teach hundreds of students and trainees. All this was done before any investigations such as X-rays, scans and blood tests were ordered.

Every morning the house surgeon, the head nurse and I would talk with our patients on our ward rounds. We spent time explaining their treatment and answering questions. We got to know much about them as individuals. Those strung up in their beds for three to four months we got to know exceptionally well.

Then there were the consultant ward rounds. The whole orthopaedic team – two consultant surgeons, a house surgeon, the chief nurse and I – would troop up to each patient. The consultant would pick up the X-ray films at the end of the bed and hold them up to the window to check the type of injury or disease and the fractured bones as we crowded round to look. My work would be assessed: the sufficiency of fixation of any hardware I had inserted; the alignment of the affected limb or spine; the length of the affected long bones. The two consultants would then confer and decide on future treatment. Occasionally, away from the patients, I would be gently told how I could have done better.

John Cullen had an infectious enthusiasm for knee surgery. I was fascinated to see the results with a series of patients in whom he had implanted an early design of a knee replacement prosthesis. These patients suffered from osteoarthritis, also called degenerative joint disease. This leads to the deterioration and eventually ulceration of articular cartilage, the tissue that covers the ends of bones where they articulate at joints. It has been known for over 250 years that such cartilage, when damaged, has little healing ability. As a famous Scottish physician, William Hunter, said in 1743: 'ulcerated cartilage is a troublesome disease' and 'when destroyed, it is not recovered'.

Joining the Herd

Normal cartilage is nourished by both the blood vessels in the underlying bone and the fluid inside the joint, which is made by the joint's lining. This lubricated bearing surface offers less frictional resistance than an ice skate gliding on ice and also acts as a shock absorber. When cartilage is damaged or worn, the underlying bone is exposed. Because bone has a nerve supply, it becomes painful when subjected to friction. Deterioration of cartilage is usually age-related, but it can also be the result of injury or another kind of joint disease included under the general term 'arthritis'.

For a long time, fusion was the operation of last resort for major pain and disability from a destroyed knee. This operation removed unhealthy cartilage that had not already been destroyed and fixed the denuded bone ends together with metal implants. In time, with a bit of luck, the two bones would unite. The outcome was a completely stiff knee that some patients understandably hated. The advent of artificial knee joint replacements, which retained knee motion, was a vast improvement. I was lucky: these devices, which caused a revolution in the treatment of osteoarthritis of the knee, were just coming into use when I became a trainee orthopaedic specialist.

I fused a knee of only one of my patients. Merv was a 37-year-old sheep and beef farmer; weather-beaten, suntanned and tough-looking. When he walked through the door of my clinic he was limping heavily, getting off his right leg quicker than his left. I could tell he was doing this to reduce pain in that leg.

'I've got this really crook right knee,' he said. 'I can't even sleep properly.'

He told me he'd had an infection somewhere around his right knee joint when he was a child and had been on antibiotics for a couple of months. According to his mother, the bug had been staphylococcus. He rolled up his trousers and showed me the scar.

I asked him how he'd been after that. 'I was mainly okay at school,' he said. 'I played rugby 'til I was about 20. It wasn't too bad for years, just used to swell up after a hard day out on the farm. But in the last six months I've been on painkillers. They don't work anymore now. I can't do the exercises the physio showed me – my knee's too sore and stiff. I have to use my quad bike most of the time. When I get off, it feels like I'm walking on broken glass.'

I examined his knee. It was swollen, deformed and stiff. X-rays showed there was no space between the bones – that meant no cartilage. And worse, the bones were wearing away because of years of bone-on-bone friction.

I told him we needed to operate. The choice was between stiffening the knee or putting in an artificial knee. A knee replacement seemed risky. Bacteria can live in a bone for decades after an infection has been treated and can become activated by surgery. Deep bacterial infection, when established around a large foreign body like a knee prosthesis, is difficult to eradicate and can result in amputation.

I consulted my colleagues. The consensus was that I should fuse the knee and not risk sepsis. The operation resulted in a firmly healed fusion. I was pleased but Merv didn't like it one bit. 'I've got to tell you, doctor, I wish we had taken the risk and gone for an artificial joint,' he told me in a follow-up consultation. I never performed another knee fusion.

Another patient came to me with a knee that had been fused by another surgeon. Hugh, a 62-year-old accountant, had sustained a serious injury to his knee years before. The surgeon had fixed the fractured bone with screws and a plate. Hugh had subsequently developed an infection so the metal had had to be removed. This time the surgeon had fused the destroyed joint.

'This so-called cure is worse than the disease I had,' he told me. 'I can't sit or drive properly with my leg stuck out in front of me. My heel kills me with pain from the pressure on it. I can't bend the knee to relieve it. I want you to take my leg off.'

I was most uncomfortable. Our job as doctors is to save limbs where at all possible. Rightly or wrongly, we equate amputation with failure. Up to this point I had amputated limbs only when there was no alternative. This man's limb was well-aligned and the fusion was sound.

We talked at length. I explained that an artificial leg fitted to a leg amputated above the knee was not very efficient. The muscles driving the artificial leg waste even more and the leg tires easily. I told him he would still have a limp. There might also be skin abrasions where the artificial leg was attached to the thigh. And more operations to refashion an ill-fitting stump.

I sent him to talk to above-knee amputees and limb-fitting experts at the Wellington Artificial Limb Service. After he had done so, he was still insistent. His wife, whom I interviewed separately with his permission, was the same so I reluctantly agreed.

I saw him again months later and inquired how he was getting on with his artificial leg. 'Do you like it better than your stiff knee?' I said. 'Not much,' he replied. 'It's a real struggle.'

From the late 1960s, hip replacements began to transform lives. Their success led surgeons to attempt knee replacements. But whereas the hip joint is a simple ball-and-socket, the knee is complex. Achieving a design for a prosthesis that would last without loosening was difficult and comparatively slow.

I saw my first knee prostheses in the mid-1970s. They were simple metal hinges, with extensions (stems) implanted and fixed with cement into the canals of the femur above and the tibia below. They often failed as the stems were forced to move more than the fixation to the bones could withstand. The hinge design ignored normal knee motion, in which the bending and straightening of the knee is accompanied by rotation, and rolling and sliding of the bones on each other. Understanding this led to changes in design and increasing success.

The knee replacements I helped John Cullen implant were not hinged. Rather, they effectively 'relined' the knee: highly polished metal on the femur above and high-density plastic on the tibia below. This made for lower friction, some rotation, and more normal mechanics. They were poor replicas and some loosened with time, but they were a big improvement on the hinge design.

Working with John, I also became interested in common and potentially disabling knee injuries. Two causes are sporting accidents (mostly soft-tissue injuries) and less commonly high-energy car crashes (more often bone fractures). Car vs. pedestrian accidents ended up with only one winner. The knee is at about the same height above the ground as the front bumper of most cars, so the collision can markedly rearrange the anatomy of one or both knees.

Direct blows to the knee are encouraged in contact sport. I was taught by my rugby coaches: 'Go low. The bigger they are, the harder they fall.' This advice is guaranteed to produce a rich harvest of knee injuries.

But there can also be non-contact knee injuries. Strong ligament-like structures hold the kneecap in place. A twist in which the upper body moves inwards and the foot is planted and rotates outwards – the common 'cutting' manoeuvre used by ball players – can rip these structures and dislocate the kneecap.

The accepted wisdom was that the medial ligament, the strap-like one on the inner side of the knee, was the commonest ligament injury and the cause of most knee weaknesses. As a trainee, the only surgery I saw to a knee ligament was to repair a torn medial.

In knees where ligament damage was not deemed severe enough to need surgery, and for blood-filled knees without a specific diagnosis, we would encase the limb in a plaster cast with the knee completely straight, usually for six weeks. By the time the cast was removed, the muscles would have become severely wasted. It would take months of exercises supervised by physiotherapists to regain muscle bulk and strength and to stretch shortened soft tissues and restore mobility. Many of the blood-filled knees would have had an ACL rupture, a fact that almost always eluded us.

Over my 50-year career the concept of rest, once prescribed for many orthopaedic conditions, has been turned on its head. The body's locomotor system is designed, unsurprisingly, for locomotion; it does not like too much rest. It is estimated that for 99.9 percent of the time that homo sapiens have been around, our modus operandi for survival has been hunting and gathering. Our ancestors lived in small bands, moving frequently in search of food. Studies of the bones of pre-agricultural humans have shown they were up to 20 percent heavier and stronger than ours. We modern humans can survive with little daily physical exercise, but if we challenge our bones more they will strengthen and the same with our muscles. Conversely, if we do little exercise our muscles will shrink and calcium flee our bones. Keep joints immobilised for a long time and they stiffen.

Bed rest for lower back pain, broken bones, injured joints and torn soft tissues has now been largely abandoned. We fix more fractures and joint instabilities early with surgery to allow our patients to safely exercise. We immobilise joints for as short a time as possible beyond the period necessary for healing. We keep patients in hospital for briefer periods. All these measures reduce recovery time. Improved fixation devices and other technology have helped this transformation, but the main driver has been knowledge of the benefits of early mobilisation: patients are helped both physically and psychologically.

13.

Going It Alone

As I gained experience as an orthopaedic registrar, I increasingly performed surgery with the assistance and guidance of the consultants. Later, I was left to operate entirely on my own; the boss would be in the tearoom, available to assist if need be. Eventually, I would perform surgery when the consultant had left the hospital at the end of his operating list.

It had become obvious that the current methods of treatment were not working for many injured knees. Our biggest deficiency was our ignorance of the knee's complex mechanics and the interaction of the four main ligaments, particularly one rather small one.

Blood and Bone

A common injury is a torn meniscus. There are two menisci. These wedge-shaped pads lie on either side of the knee between the femur and the tibia and are made of strong fibrous tissue – so-called 'fibro-cartilage'. Either meniscus can tear when there is a sudden twisting of a weight-bearing knee. A loose piece can then get pinched and cause pain, swelling or catching. A large fragment may jam the joint, making the knee lock, unable to straighten. In other cases, the knee may give way. Menisci in older people lose resilience and can tear with a minor injury. Sometimes the person is not even aware they have had an injury.

Surgery for a torn meniscus was either removal of the loose piece or, more often, cutting out the whole meniscus. We would make an incision of several centimetres in the front of the knee, to one side of the knee cap. This 'open' operation was followed by several days on pain relief medicines in a hospital.

Many tears were confined to the back of the meniscus and difficult, even impossible, to see from the incision in the front of the knee. Sometimes, when the symptoms the patient described seemed to indicate a tear, we would just assume the tear was present and remove the meniscus. I had a sinking feeling whenever a removed meniscus showed no tear. We had just removed a normal structure. Fortunately, this was rare.

Our knowledge of the function of the meniscus was

woefully inadequate. Occasionally, at the time of an initial surgery, or later if symptoms continued, we might make a second incision – this time at the back of the knee – to remove a chunk of meniscus not removable from the front. The meniscus was often wrongly blamed for the ongoing symptoms. We were sometimes ripping out a valuable and important knee structure. A torn anterior cruciate ligament was often the actual cause of the symptoms. Fortunately, I was about to learn a better way of doing things.

Also on the boss's team was Bill Gillespie, a fulltime consultant. Bill became a valuable mentor. Whenever I had to deal with complex cases I would call him rather than the boss, who worked in the public hospital only part-time, hence he didn't have to get involved with his patients' care at nights or on his weekends on-call.

This was the way things had been forever. Initially many hospital specialists were 'honorary', working part-time in public hospitals as a service to the community. Later, although the consultants were paid, the arrangement stayed the same. A young aspiring doctor would cover the acute after-hours work while the chief advised from home. Few senior consultants would come into the hospital to help unless there was a major emergency. We were reluctant to call them in anyway, fiercely determined to cope on our own. In retrospect, this was probably to the disadvantage of both us and our patients.

Blood and Bone

In the mid '70s we junior doctors went public. We arranged a full-page ad in an Auckland newspaper to inform the public that they might be treated by exhausted doctors. Over a photo of an operating theatre, we compared the rates of pay of the various workers around the table. They included junior doctor-surgeons, their medical assistants, nurses and orderlies. The hourly rate of pay for us 80-hour weekend doctors looked pathetic alongside the pay of those who worked normal eight-hour days. Our argument was not primarily about money: we reasoned that if hospital administrators had to pay us a better hourly rate they would be disinclined to work us so long at a stretch.

Incensed by our activism and the newspaper ad, one senior doctor wrote a letter to the newspaper excoriating us. The boss used another method, threatening the future careers of juniors who spoke out. There were warning signs that this highly regarded doctor was into power in a big way. When I was selected for training in orthopaedics, he had taken Pamela aside at a social function. 'You know that your husband is joining a group of surgeons who have a lot of influence on those in political power,' he said.

A woman at the New Zealand Medical Association organised for a newspaper journalist to interview wives of junior doctors about the impact of working hours on our families. The article was accompanied by a photo showing our wives and children. The night it appeared I arrived home to hear that the boss had phoned. 'Are you the Pamela Tregonning whose photo appeared in the paper among a group of junior doctors' wives?' he said. 'Yes,' Pamela replied. 'That's all I want to know,' he said and hung up.

Alarmed, I rang a fellow registrar, whose wife had also been in the photo. He reported that the boss had also rung and threatened him. 'Firstly, I won't have you work with me,' he had said. 'Secondly, I'm not going to support you in an overseas job. And thirdly, I'm going to make sure you don't pass your final fellowship examination.' The fellowship was essential to gain a consultant job in New Zealand and my colleague had not yet sat the examination. I had, so the boss couldn't threaten me with the same thing.

With some trepidation, I phoned him. It was about ten p.m. I'd never before rung him at this hour. 'Sorry to ring you this late, but I want to discuss the issue that prompted you to ring and speak to my wife tonight,' I said. 'I gather you have also spoken with my colleague. Can we please meet with you tomorrow?'

He agreed and stated a time and place. At the meeting I assured him that our main argument was with the hospital authorities. This was only half true but I felt it wiser not to highlight his opposition to our attempts to improve our working conditions. My career was at stake. I was running scared, despite my outward bravado.

We seemed to settle him: he didn't carry out his threats.

My colleague passed his fellowship exam and went on to practise in the United States, never to work as a consultant in New Zealand. Ironically, the boss later became chair of the NZMA, the organisation that had helped us by setting up the newspaper interview.

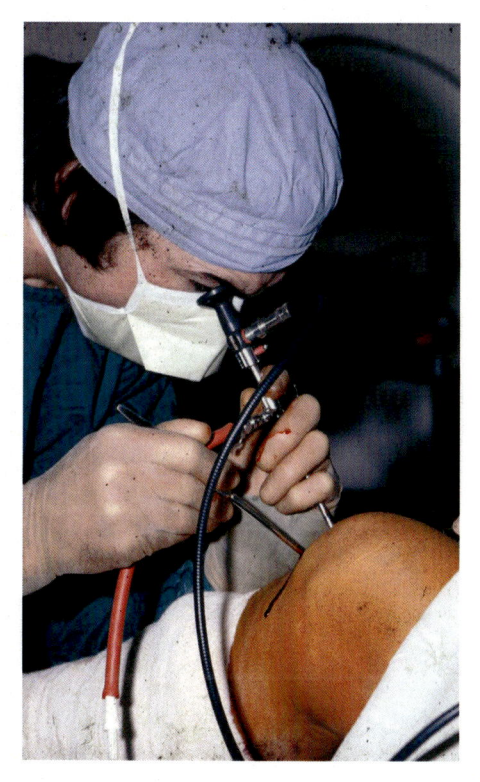

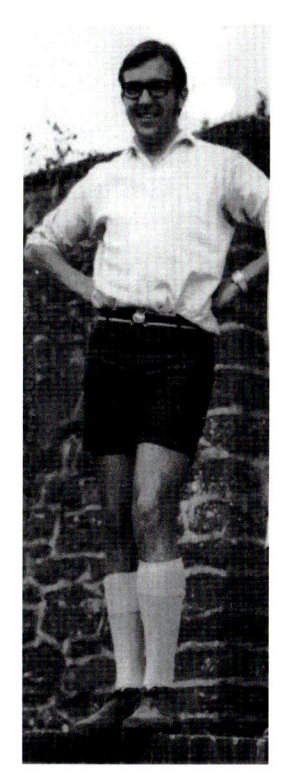

Above: Early scope NB hygiene; (right) Russell Tregonning in Plymouth, 1971.
Below: Ship's doctor en route to London on *Majestic* 1970, Capetown.

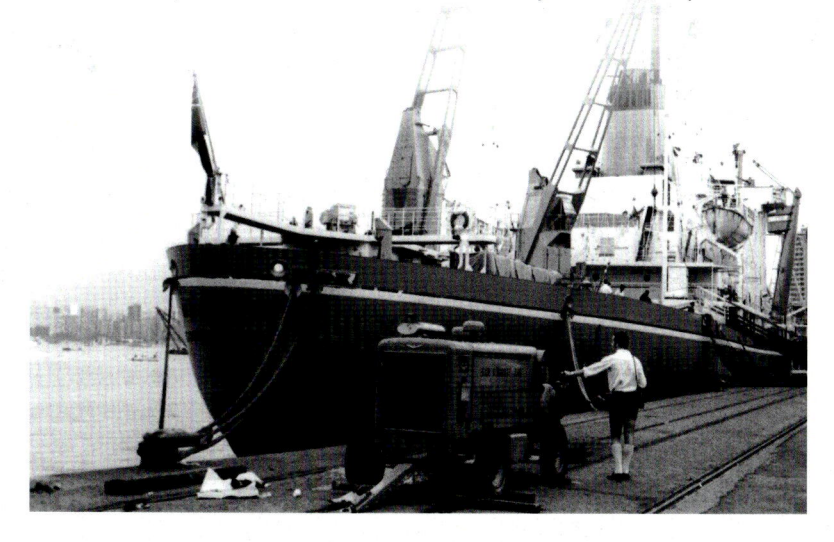

Knee anatomy

Front view

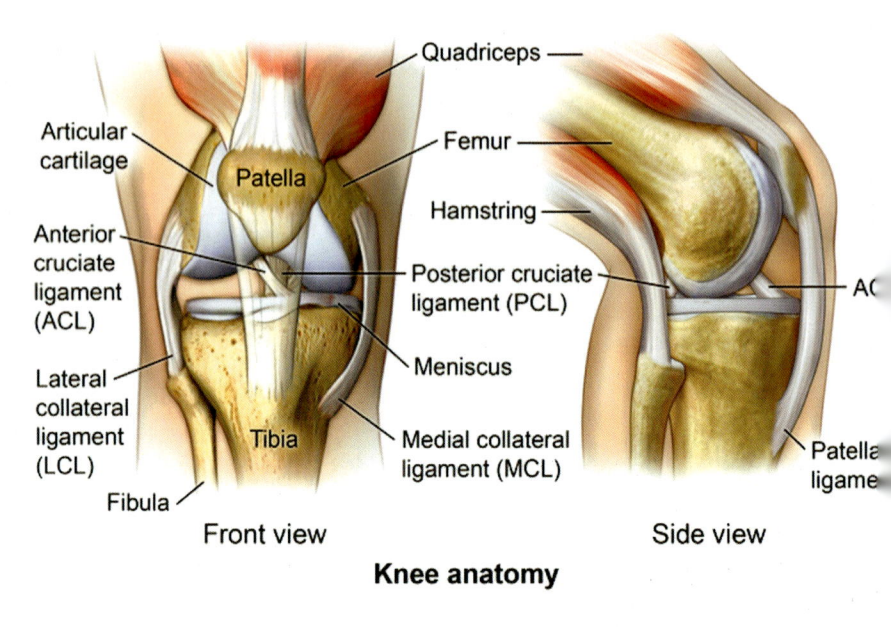

- Quadriceps
- Articular cartilage
- Patella
- Femur
- Anterior cruciate ligament (ACL)
- Hamstring
- Posterior cruciate ligament (PCL)
- Meniscus
- Lateral collateral ligament (LCL)
- Tibia
- Medial collateral ligament (MCL)
- Fibula

Side view

- AC
- Patella ligame

Instruments used in total knee replacement. Photograph: Stuff Limited.

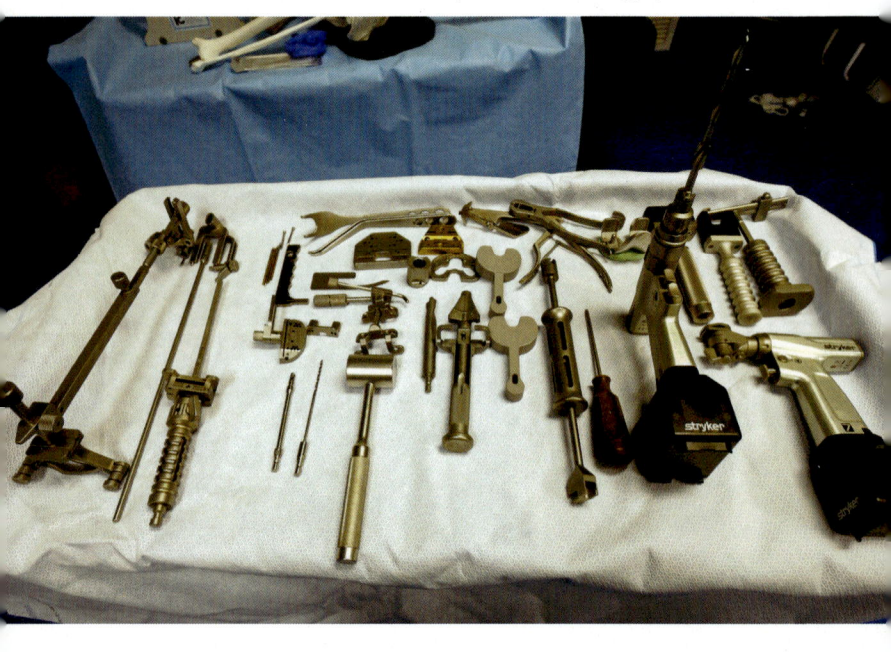

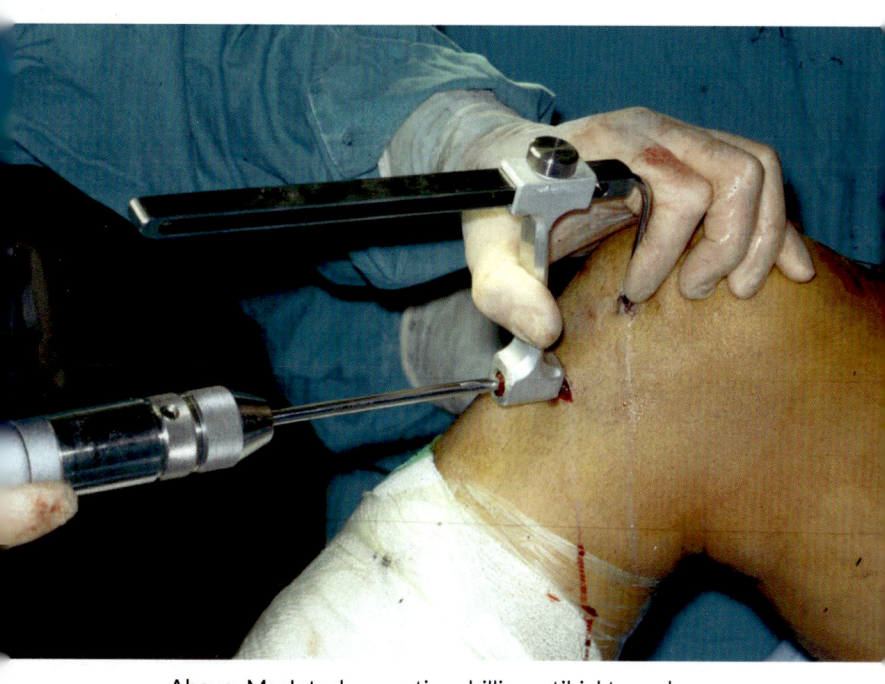

Above: MacIntosh operation drilling a tibial tunnel.
Below: Donor strip of tissue.

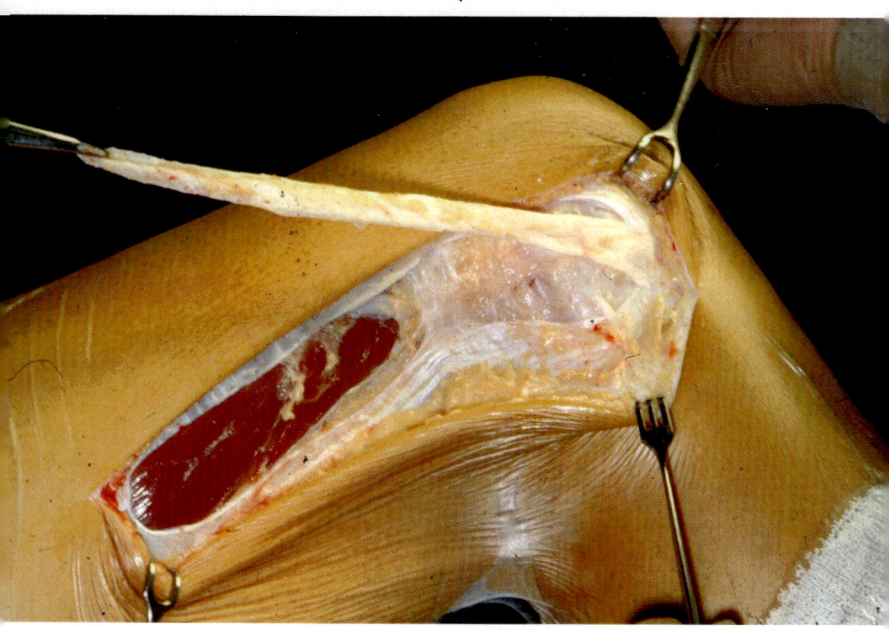

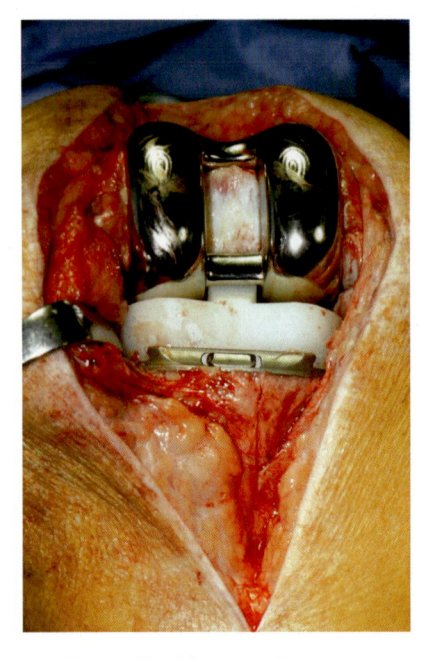

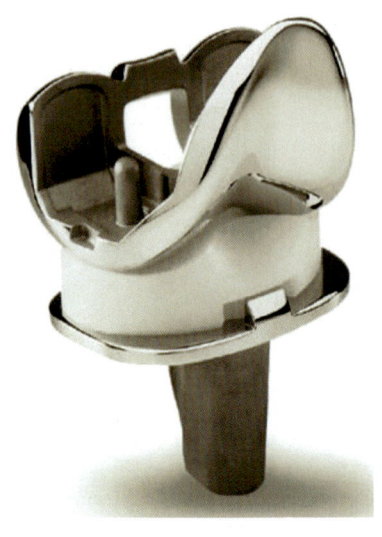

Above: Total knee replacement at surgery; (right) Total knee front view.
Below: Oxford uni normal X-ray side view; (right) Oxford uni front view.

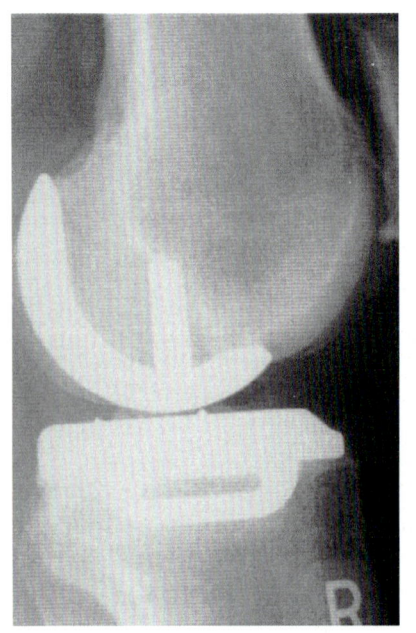

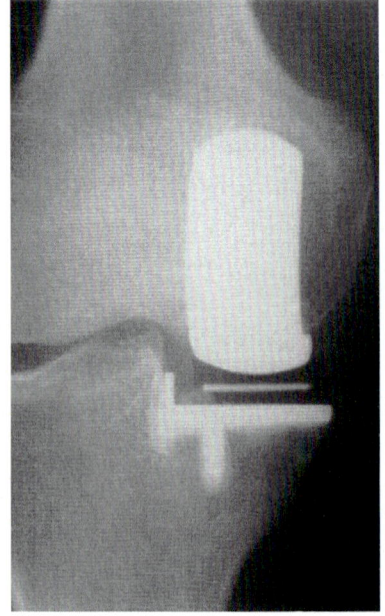

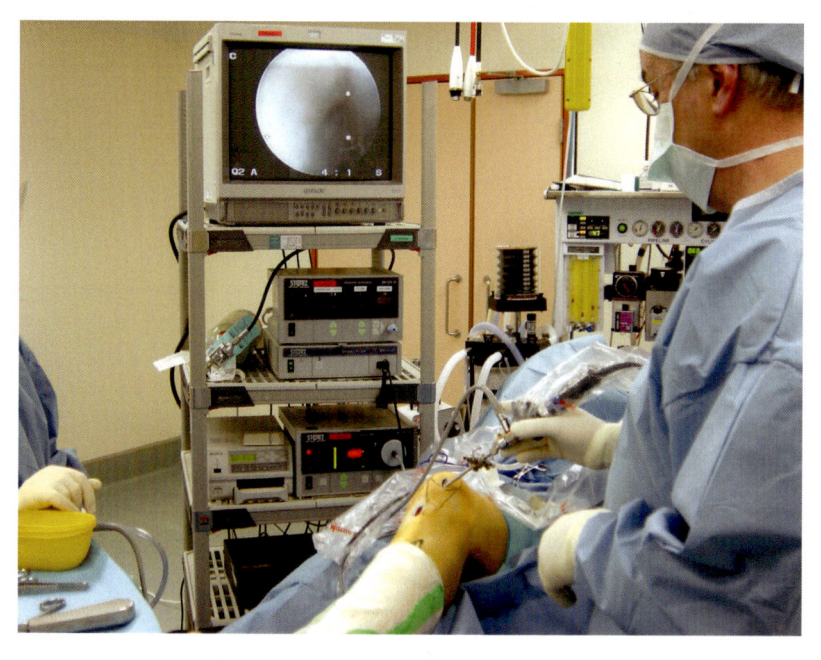

Above: Arthroscopic ACLR using B-PT-B.
Below: 'The Nisbo' (the wire being pointed to by the forceps).

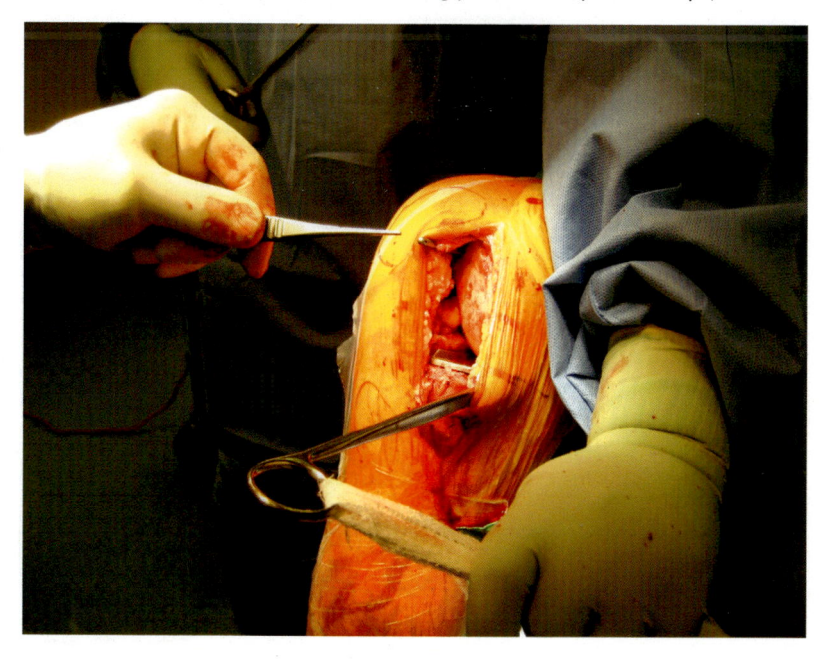

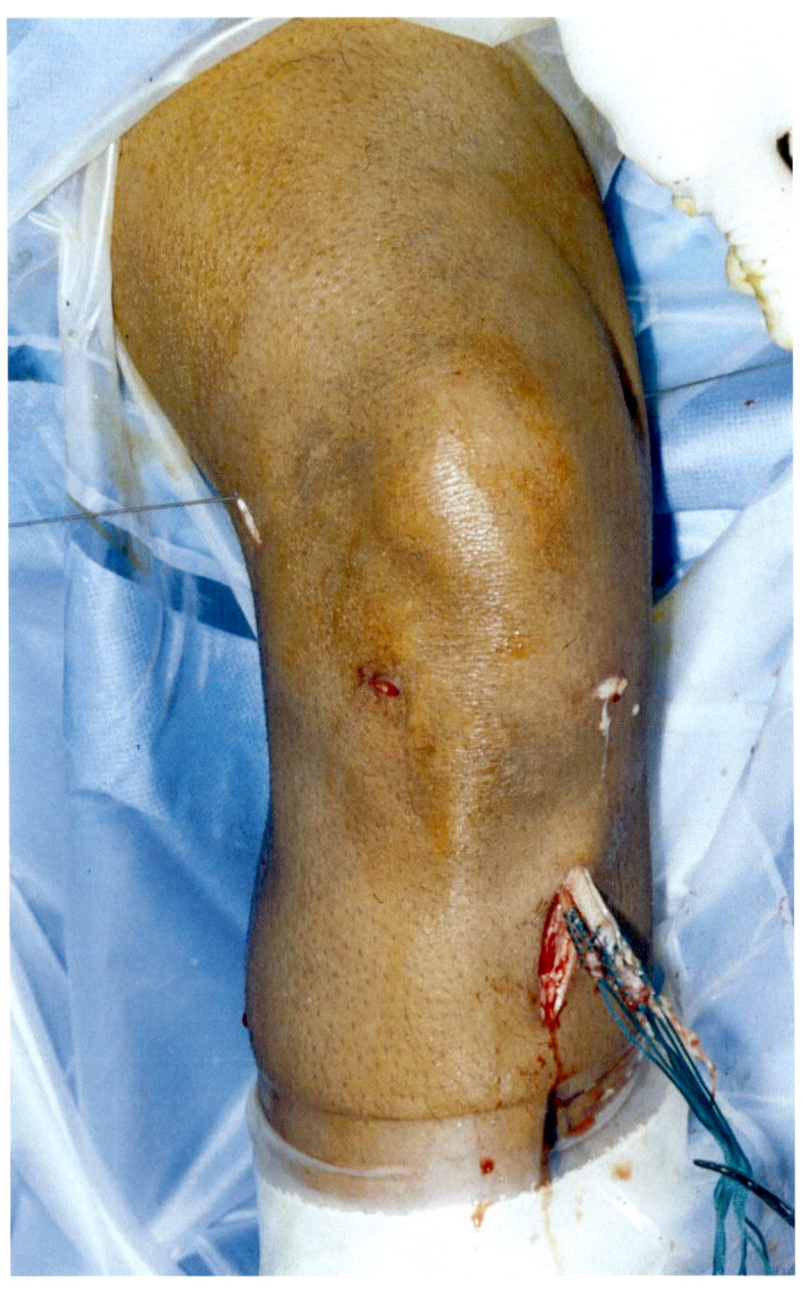

Arthroscopic hamstring ACL reconstruction

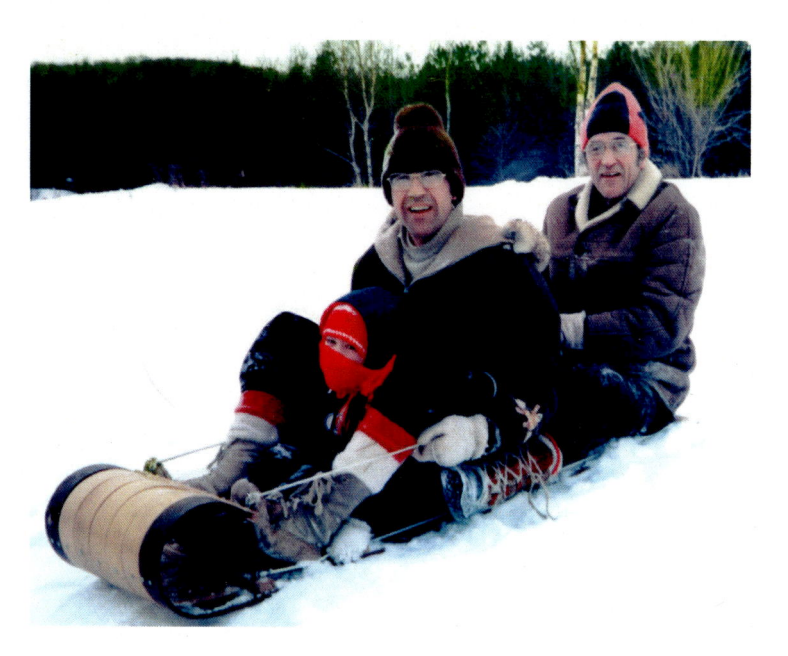

Above: David MacIntosh, Russell and Mark Tregonning, 1976, Canada.

Below: Back from left: Camilla Tregonning-Duff, Andrew Duff, Russell Tregonning, Pamela Tregonning. Middle: Ella Tregonning-Duff.
Front from left: Riley Tregonning-Duff, Mark Tregonning.

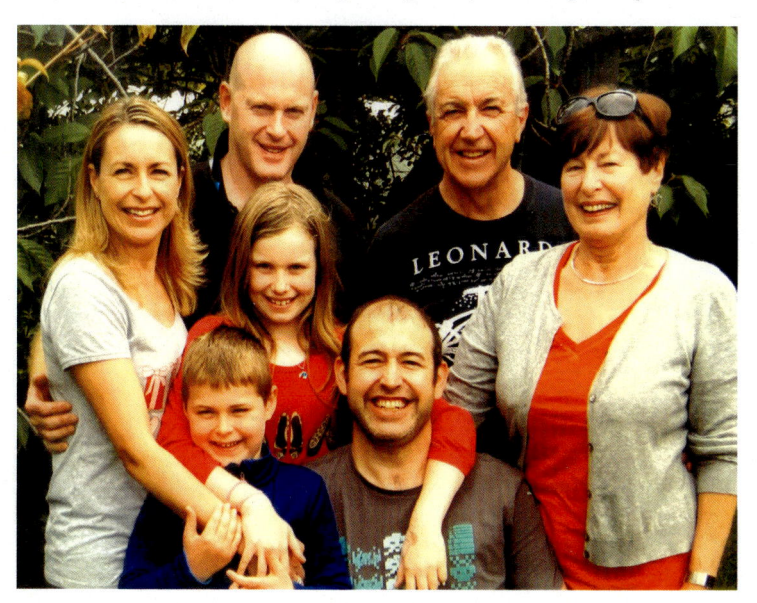

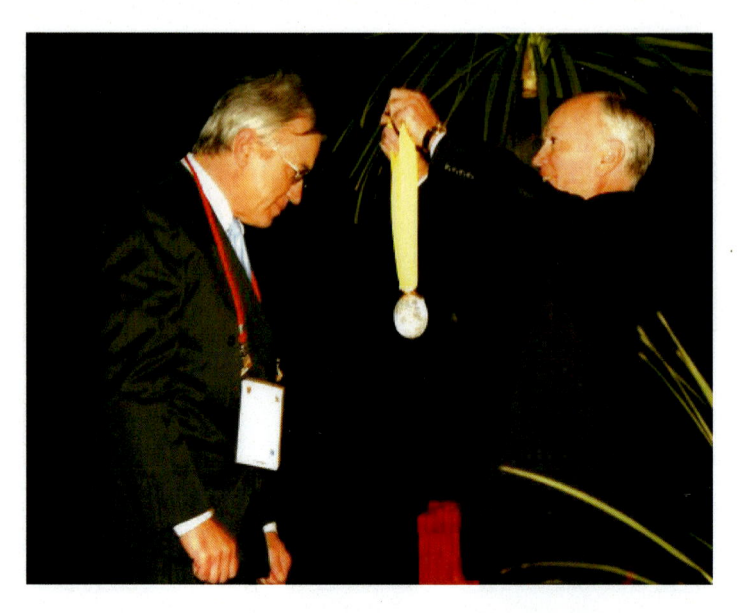

Above: Past NZOA President Garnet Tregonning and new President Russell Tregonning, 2005.

Below: Russell Tregonning at Wise Response launch, Dunedin 2013.

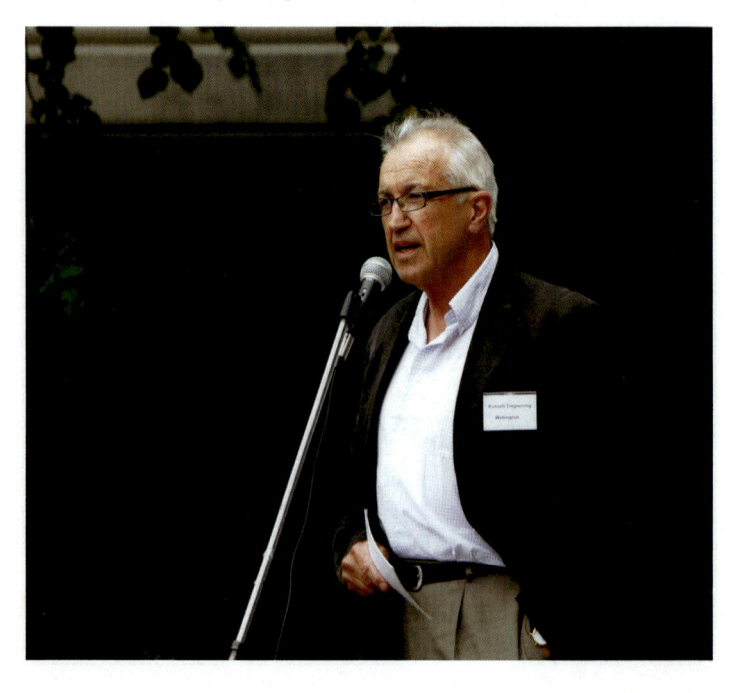

14.

In Mackenzie Country

ASPIRING ORTHOPAEDIC SURGEONS IN New Zealand spend time overseas in large orthopaedic units to hone their skills before taking up positions as senior consultants. Garnet had spent several years in Toronto, where the hospitals had a reputation for orthopaedic excellence. He encouraged me to apply and I was lucky enough to get a fellowship, partly on the strength of the reference the boss had given me before our altercation.

I needed cash for our flights to Toronto and accommodation once we were there. Two months before we were to depart, I saw an advertisement for a locum to help the sole GP in Twizel, Neil McKenzie. Twizel is a small town in the Mackenzie country, ringed to the west by the Southern Alps and named after James Mackenzie, a sheep-stealing outlaw and no relation to Neil. Twizel was run by the Ministry of Works and had been built mainly to house workers on the large Upper Waitaki hydroelectric dam projects between the great lakes. At its peak, about the time I was there, the population was roughly 6000. The two closest centres with hospitals of any size were Ōamaru and Timaru, both around 150 kilometres away.

I had serious doubts about my suitability for a job in such a far-flung place; my old bête noir, obstetrics, was uppermost in my mind. I spoke to Neil on the phone. After introductions I got down to the nitty-gritty. 'Neil, I love the sound of the job in a part of the country I know well, but I have no obstetric experience that I'm willing to tell you about.'

'Russell, that won't be any kind of problem,' he said. 'I'll be living in the house next door. I nearly did my fellowship in O&G and I'll be comfortable to help you any time. Just call me and I'll be there. We have a huge number of orthopaedic injuries with the dam workers. You'll be in your element down here.'

I discussed it with Pamela. We'd be close to our southern relatives and particularly both our parents, who had Central Otago holiday homes. Despite my professional misgivings, we decided to go.

In Mackenzie Country

The setting was spectacular. The Ben Ohau range dominated the view to the west. Not far away to the north was Aoraki/Mt Cook, New Zealand's highest mountain; on a clear day it was visible through the window of my office. It was also cold, with beautiful hoar frosts. Wet clothes on the line were stiff as a board within an hour or two. But there were menacing sights in the town centre: every woman seemed to be of child-bearing age and many bulged threateningly. When a woman was admitted to the small maternity annex in labour, I borrowed Neil's obstetrics textbook and read furiously.

For a while deliveries went well, thanks to a lot of help from my midwife colleagues. But then what I had feared happened – an obstetric nightmare in an alpine paradise. When Neil had told me he would be around to help with obstetric cases, what he had forgotten to tell me was that every second weekend he would be skiving off into the countryside in his vintage car.

On one such weekend a woman in labour arrived. Early on everything seemed to be going all right, but as time wore on and progress slowed the patient became distressed. So did I. It had become obvious that the baby's head was stuck sideways: the mother's cervix was fully dilated, which usually means birth is imminent, but the head was jammed across her pelvis and wouldn't budge.

I was completely out of my depth, with no idea what

to do. In a lather, I phoned the obstetrics specialist at Timaru Hospital, who said, 'Put plenty of fluid through the drip, give maximum pain relief, and get her down here as soon as you can.'

I called for an ambulance. In two hours the mother was in capable hands. The baby was born with a forceps delivery. I decided then and there that I should never again be let near a woman in labour.

The price women pay for our upright stance as humans is a narrow pelvis. And our babies have disproportionately large heads compared to those of mammals that get around on all fours. Big head through narrow pelvis makes human childbirth painful and hazardous.

A true miracle is the huge decline in maternal mortality – death in pregnancy or within six weeks of childbirth. My paternal great-grandmother, Emma Gridgeman, died in 1906, aged 30, just after delivering her tenth child. The cause was puerperal sepsis: severe infection arising from the birth canal. This was then the most common cause of maternal death. In the *New Zealand Journal of History* in 2017, academic Maureen Molloy recorded in an article entitled 'Maternal and Infant Mortality, 1870 – 1930' that the New Zealand maternal mortality rate in 1906 was about four per thousand births. In 2017 it was 44 times lower.

In Mackenzie Country

Glentanner Station, about 60 kilometres from Twizel, is reputedly the highest sheep station in New Zealand. One Saturday the phone rang. 'Doc, get down here to the police station pronto. A man is bleeding badly up at Glentanner.'

I picked up bags of plasma and saline from the surgery and hurried to the police station down the road. Soon I was in a police car speeding up the Mt Cook road. When we got to Glentanner we found an elderly man lying on the ground in a pool of blood. I bent over him. 'Can you hear me,' I said. He didn't reply. 'Can you hear me?' I repeated. Silence.

There was a tear in the man's blood-soaked trousers over his groin. I checked his pulse. It was weak and fast. Several men were standing around. I said to one of them, 'Here, push this pad firmly over the groin and hold it there to stop the bleeding.'

While I tapped urgently at the man's elbow crease, found a vein and inserted a plasma drip, the station owner told me what had happened. There was a pet tahr that hung out at the station. When the man had bent over to stroke the animal, it had butted him in the groin.

Plasma is the part of blood left after red cells that contain the pigment haemoglobin have been removed. It is yellowish, stored in plastic bags and can be given to patients through an IV drip, followed by saline to increase the blood volume, without waiting to find out the person's blood type. For patients with severe blood loss, it can save lives as it did in this case. The deer antlers hanging high up in the shed made a handy stand on which to hang the bag of plasma.

After I had squeezed the first bag of plasma into his vein, the man came around. 'Where am I?' he asked, dazed. An ambulance soon arrived and he was taken to Timaru Hospital for blood transfusion and surgical repair of his femoral artery. I heard that he had an uneventful recovery.

I congratulated myself. It seemed that as long as no obstetrics was involved, I could cope with emergencies quite well. But my confidence was premature. The next emergency case in which I was involved would not go at all well.

15.

Toronto Finishing School

IN JULY 1976, PAMELA AND I, with our five-year-old daughter and three-year-old son, packed our bags and headed for Toronto. We arrived in the middle of a hot humid Canadian summer and rented a house in Scarborough, an outer suburb. Most people in the neighbourhood were away on holiday. To make matters worse, I immediately rushed off and worked long hours in the central city hospital. Early each morning I would make a two-train journey to work. More than once I fell asleep exhausted and missed my stop. I spent little time with my young family.

Toronto was a leading centre for orthopaedics in the English-speaking world and much was expected of aspiring surgeons. Garnet told me the senior surgeon who taught him had proudly said that Toronto graduates would have their qualification 'branded on their backside'.

I was to find out the truth of this. Toronto was like another planet. I was not used to the rushed ward rounds at six-thirty in the morning. One of my seniors told me he liked them because the patients were still half asleep and didn't ask questions. I preferred our laidback New Zealand style. I enjoyed relating to patients and explaining the detail of our treatments fully. The practice culture was frenetic and high-pressure from early in the morning until late at night, often with no lunch. I quickly lost weight. I began to think that had I been Canadian I would never have chosen orthopaedics.

My practice was little supervised. As well as assisting seniors, I had a few minor operating lists and clinics of my own. In addition, we fellows were expected to involve ourselves in clinical research on our seniors' patients, exploring aspects of diagnosis or treatment. We were to research the topic then review patients, assess results and write papers. As usual, I bit off more than I could chew. I finished a time-consuming but ultimately rewarding research project but left two others unfinished. Why did I think I could do three?

Luckily, though, I came under the influence of two pioneer giants of knee surgery. Both were patient, kind men who generously shared their skills and knowledge. Studying under them had not been my original idea, which had been to train at Toronto's celebrated Hospital for Sick Children under its well-known chief of paediatric orthopaedic surgery, Robert Salter. But when I arrived in Toronto, I learnt that all fellows' jobs at the hospital were filled.

I was offered a 12-month fellowship at Toronto General with a surgeon team of my choice. Garnet had shown me an unpublished article by David MacIntosh, an orthopaedic surgeon at the hospital, in which he described a novel examination technique he had worked out to test the stability of injured athletes' knees. I couldn't understand the concepts, but I was intrigued. Everyone I spoke to in Toronto referred to MacIntosh with affection as Mac. I signed up to work on a team that included him. The next 12 months were to have a profound influence on my career.

David MacIntosh was an energetic surgeon, researcher and lateral thinker. He looked at knee joint problems in a highly original way and devised and performed new operations. He was by then in his early sixties. I was amazed at his work ethic. After a full day at the hospital he would walk over to the University of Toronto's Hart House clinic for injured athletes, which he had established in the 1950s. Now known as the David L. MacIntosh Sport Medicine Clinic and in a different venue, it is thought to be the world's oldest dedicated sports medicine facility.

I sometimes helped Mac at Hart House. Modern photos show a well-lit, smart facility, a far cry from the dark cavern in which we worked. If I or one of the other fellows wasn't there to help, Mac carried out the work on his own. There was only one technician, so Mac mostly did his own plastering.

It was at Hart House that he developed his ideas about the injured knee. Sometimes he would treat acute injuries suffered close by, even in the same building. Once, when he was busy plastering a broken limb, I was called to the gym adjacent to the clinic. 'Can you come quickly. A gymnast has fallen and his elbow is out of shape.' I asked the distressed athlete how the injury had happened. 'I fell on my hand,' he said, 'and felt the elbow bones come apart.'

The man's elbow shouted dislocation. I quickly manipulated the joint without anaesthetic. The body's response to an injury like this is to release hormones that dampen pain. The man hardly winced as I jerked the elbow back into place with a satisfying 'thunk'. The elbow looked like an elbow again.

On one of my first days on the ward, Mac took me to see a patient and instructed: 'Please take a history, examine the patient's knee and make a diagnosis.' Six months previously the young man had suffered an injury at football and been forced to leave the field. Within an hour, his knee had swelled up. Over the following weeks the swelling had settled but he had continued to suffer intermittent pain with disabling instability. He had tried to return to football but had experienced multiple episodes where his knee had collapsed, dropping him to the ground. More swelling had followed each episode.

I performed my usual knee examination. 'He has probably torn his medial meniscus,' I said.

'And what about his ligaments?' Mac said.

The ligaments appeared normal. To test the ACL I performed the 'anterior drawer test' I had been taught. This involved trying to pull the tibia forward on the femur with the knee at 90 degrees, like pulling the drawer of a chest of drawers. If the ACL is intact, there is usually only a few millimetres of movement. I performed the same test on the uninjured knee. Both had the same amount of movement. I judged the ACL to be intact.

Mac took hold of the knee. I'd never seen anything like it. The anterior drawer test he did was slight, about 20 to 30 degrees of flexion. This mimicked the position the knee would have been in when the athlete twisted and it collapsed. This result was completely different. The amount of 'drawer' Mac obtained on the injured knee with slight flexion was abnormally increased compared to the other knee. A light bulb went on in my head. Of course, we should examine the knee at the position it was in when injured. This was less painful for the patient as well.

Mac said, 'Let me show you the lateral pivot shift sign.' He then did the test he had described in his paper. Manipulating the slightly bent knee again, he twisted the lower leg internally while pushing it forward. The knee fell apart. The man cried, 'That's it! The bones moved out of place. That's what my knee does when it collapses.'

I shared his eureka moment. Mac was reproducing the forces acting on the knee when the ACL ruptured. In New Zealand we followed the teaching of Ian Smillie, a celebrated Scottish knee injury expert and the author of our standard knee textbooks. For 'internal derangements of the knee' Smillie discounted the ACL and blamed the meniscus. I realised that I and my colleagues back home were missing ACL injuries in droves. The conventional tests we had been taught were near useless.

The bony anatomy of the knee appears unlikely to hold up under stress. The two longest bones in the body are stuck, one on top of the other. The outer femur is convex from front to back, as is the outer tibia with which it articulates, ball-on-ball. With such incongruity, only soft tissues and muscle action hold the bones correctly together.

These have to resist the huge forces generated during running, twisting, jumping and decelerating. The main non-muscular restraints are the ligaments, thin ropes joining the bones. The most often injured of those resisting rotation in the outside knee compartment is the comparatively weak anterior cruciate ligament.

The ACL commonly tears in ball sports that involve leaping, and when a running athlete suddenly changes direction. Most of these injuries are non-contact – there is no direct blow to the knee. Athletes in non-ball sports that involve twisting or leaping, such as skiing, dancing and gymnastics, are also at risk. Direct blows or severe twisting can injure other ligaments as well; contact tackling sports such as rugby and rugby league may cause injuries to more than one knee ligament.

Netball is the most played women's sport in New Zealand. It involves a lot of aerial acrobatics, but players have to come back to earth. Female players rupture the ACL at several times the rate of males in the same sport. The rules of netball state: 'Once a player has landed with the ball, the first landed foot is called the grounded foot and must either stay on the ground or in the air until the ball is passed on.' Landing on one leg and suddenly stopping, combined with a twist, puts the ACL at risk.

The knee with a torn ACL only partially dislocates and immediately snaps back into place. Although poleaxed to the ground and sometimes in a lot of pain, the player can usually take some weight on the knee afterwards, albeit with a painful limp. But just like my patient at the Hart House gym with the dislocated elbow, the athlete often senses that something dramatic has happened. Some patients hear a dramatic noise as the taut ACL explodes. In 2005 I treated Japanese dancer Yu Takayama, principal ballerina of the Royal New Zealand Ballet. During a solo performance on stage, Yu's knee collapsed and, as *Metro* magazine reported, 'she was forced to drag herself to the haven of the wings. The curtain fell, leaving the Aotea Centre audience shocked. ... Takayama can still hear the loud bang as the ligaments of the right knee separated.' The hormone rush at the time of injury may have saved her from immediate pain but her knee would have been painful soon afterwards. Others feel excruciating pain immediately.

Not all patients with this rupture develop symptoms of instability. Anatomical differences play a part. Well-tuned muscles can help prevent too much abnormal motion, hence the importance of major rehabilitation with muscle strengthening. But the original injury may injure menisci and smooth cartilage, and repeated episodes make these injuries more likely.

David MacIntosh used the words 'anterior cruciate ligament syndrome' to describe ACL injuries in a patient whose knee then repeatedly gives way. The result can be irreversible osteoarthritis, so he stressed the importance of making an early diagnosis and advising the patient to undertake muscle strengthening, avoid dangerous sports and consider surgical reconstruction.

Toronto Finishing School

MacIntosh had discovered the lateral pivot shift test decades before I worked with him and had devised operations to repair and later to reconstruct torn ACLs. His repair operation initially tried to sew together the two loose ends of the ligaments. This was successful only for some patients. Then he detached and rerouted a strip of tendon-like fibrous tissue on the outer thigh to strengthen the outer compartment of the knee and keep the bones in place – the 'lateral (ACL) substitution' operation.

His methods evolved over time. Later he strengthened the repair by taking the lateral strip through the back of the knee and into the joint, along the line of the sutured ACL. After some patients found instability returned, he used a stronger tendon strip from the front of the knee – the 'quadriceps-patellar tendon graft'. By the time I worked with him, he had reconstructed many knees using these novel techniques.

Some of my time was spent following up Mac's patients to assess how they were faring after their operations. Many lived far away in provincial Ontario. Pamela and I with our two small children combined exploration with business as I chased them up, questioned them and examined their knees. I presented the results at the annual meeting of the Canadian Orthopaedic Association in June 1977.

Mac's own oral presentations were sometimes quirky. At one he got a patient with a reconstructed ACL to run up and down the aisle of the lecture theatre, changing direction and stopping suddenly. My show was dry by comparison, consisting largely of slides. However, I felt a surge of pleasure when a well-known authority in the orthopaedic world said to me afterwards, 'Your presentation was the first time I really understood what Mac was on about.'

To have new thinking accepted in medicine, it is almost obligatory to publish a substantial paper in a well-known journal, but for Mac this was not a priority. He just got on with nutting out new concepts and developing ways of improving patients' lives. Ironically, Mac's pivot shift concept was first written up after a 1971 presentation by Bob Galway, a previous MacIntosh fellow, to the New Zealand Orthopaedic Association's annual scientific meeting. An abstract appeared in the *Journal of Bone and Joint Surgery* but clearly didn't set the orthopaedic world on fire. When I trained in orthopaedics in Auckland in the mid-1970s, I had neither heard nor read anything about the pivot shift.

One of David MacIntosh's most famous patients was Victoria Tennant, a principal dancer with the National Ballet of Canada. Tennant went to see him in 1977 after she had injured her knee and been told her ballet career was over. 'I told Dr MacIntosh I intend to dance again,' Tennant wrote in MacIntosh's obituary in the *Toronto Globe and*

Mail in 2013. 'He said "deal" and shook my hand. It was my left knee, which is the one needed for the pyrotechnic challenges of *Swan Lake*, one of the most daunting roles for a ballerina.'

MacIntosh transformed the dancer's life. After he operated on her knee she danced for another 12 years until retiring in 1989. 'The second half of my career was better than the first,' she wrote.

Ballerinas, although they look delicate, are tough, determined athletes. Their will to succeed makes them perfect patients on whom to perform knee surgery. They adhere to extended and vigorous rehabilitation programmes to regain the power and flexibility they need. As the *Metro* article about Yu Takayama stated: 'Many hours of swimming, weight-training, Pilates and gym work have filled her days. ... Takayama had a mental toughness. She saw the recuperation period as a chance to fix her body, away from the rigour of constant performance.'

Neither MacIntosh nor I gave these top professional ballerinas a chance to see whether their knee would give way again without surgery. We felt the risk of further injury from the pyrotechnics involved in their demanding routines was too high. Their careers were at stake. The sooner their knees were stabilised, the sooner they could dance again.

David MacIntosh did not limit his help to the normal

working week. On weekends and evenings, he helped university players in football and ice hockey teams. Occasionally I covered for him. This was a real education. I had been a lifelong rugby player, so to me Canadian football looked shambolic, with players rushing on and off the field, apparently at will. The same was true of ice hockey. I knew little of the rules of either game but that didn't matter – my job was to tend the injured.

Ice hockey is played indoors. It was fast, with loud organ music, occasionally rising to a climax, generating an exciting atmosphere. I was surprised at its brutality. There was much barging body contact as players attempted to separate an attacker from the puck, a defensive manoeuvre called 'checking'. This involved driving the shoulder, upper arm, hip and elbow to force the attacking player's body against the boards – the high side of the playing area – or onto the ice. The most common injuries were to the head and face; they included concussion and facial laceration. I sutured a number of wounds that seemed to be inflicted by a hockey stick, mostly I hoped unintentionally. The next most frequent were ligament injuries caused by blows to the side of the knee.

Mac had a reputation for absentmindedness. One story was that he walked out of the operating change-room in somebody else's shoes. In another, he took his son on a ward round one morning, forgot he had, and went home without him. As we scrubbed up for knee surgery I would observe him thinking, thinking. Although he would have examined the patient's knee thoroughly, he would suddenly leave while half-scrubbed, don gloves and go back into the operating room to re-examine the patient. Then he would re-scrub. He seemed intensely absorbed, always looking for new ways to solve a problem.

He was also a pioneer in treating arthritis of the knee with knee replacements. He used an entirely new early prototype. In his obituary in the *Globe and Mail* his son Doug MacIntosh described how this began. 'There was an experimental artificial joint prosthesis, made in Denmark, being used as an ashtray in the surgeons' lounge at the hospital. He cut it in half ... sterilised it and used it to replace the joint surface in the [woman's] knee. Without that new technique, the knee would have been fused, leaving the patient with no motion for the rest of her life.'

These early Macintosh prostheses were simply metallic discs shaped like a half moon and slipped between the bones to substitute for worn-off cartilage. Although they relieved pain, they were prone to dislocate. The next generation of prostheses were fixed to the bone with cement.

Mac became a special person in my life, unfailingly warm and supportive. In winter, he invited my family and me to his 200-acre rural property northeast of Toronto.

A keen skier, he had installed a rope tow on a hill. In thick snow, he took me and my three-year-old son Mark for a spin on his skidoo.

After leaving Toronto I contacted him each time I returned. In June 1992, almost 15 years to the day since I had first presented his work to the Canadian Orthopaedic Association, I presented my own series of MacIntosh ACL reconstructions to the Ninth Combined Meeting of the Orthopaedic Associations of the English-Speaking World in Toronto. Mac, aged 78, was in the audience. Afterwards over coffee we talked about old times and I expressed my gratitude to him. For me, it was an emotional meeting.

The fellows at Toronto General Hospital were assigned the care of the injured members of the indigent population. I gathered there were financial implications: these uninsured patients were treated free of charge, thereby attracting no surgeon fee. I was paid a salary, so no money changed hands between patient and surgeon.

One of the first of these patients for whom I was responsible had a fracture of the shaft of his thigh bone, or femur. In New Zealand, I had been schooled in the conservative British school of orthopaedics, where fractured bones were largely treated without operation. I put the man's leg in traction to restore leg line and length over a prolonged period of bed rest. The leg was supported in a primitive-looking Thomas splint, a gadget first used a century before by a Welsh surgeon, Hugh Owen Thomas.

Treatments like this, although avoiding the risks of surgery, were followed by stiff joints; patients would often need lengthy physiotherapy to mobilise their legs and build back muscle strength. Toronto had adopted the European techniques of internal fixation that had originated mainly in Switzerland. These newer methods encouraged more predictable results. Operations held broken fragments of bone securely with metallic implants. Patients were able to walk and function earlier, reducing harmful bed rest and hospital stays.

I had little knowledge of these techniques. My Canadian juniors clearly thought I had come out of the ark.

I had another bad experience treating a frail elderly woman with an open fracture of her main lower leg bone, the tibia. An 'open' fracture is one that's exposed to air through the torn overlying soft tissue and skin. Although I used the conventional treatment, thoroughly washing the wound, removing the dead tissue and prescribing high doses of penicillin, the woman developed gas gangrene. This is a feared complication brought about by bacteria that thrives in tissues deprived of blood and oxygen. Despite our vigorous treatment, the woman slowly went downhill. A nasty stench emanated from her discharging wound. I thought she would not survive amputation.

She took days to die. I was gutted at having to stand by impotently and watch.

There were other disturbing cases. I felt increasingly inadequate, inferior and depressed. I lost weight rapidly and my clothes began to hang loose on me. Decision-making became very difficult. A major stress was that I couldn't decide about what I should do after my 12 months in Toronto. Our original plan was to travel to Oxford where I would take up a further 12 month job as a Nuffield orthopaedic fellow. But an orthopaedic friend recently having completed that job warned me against doing so as the salary was low and he felt the experience not worth the effort. There would be costs and further family disruption with travel to another far-off country so, although I was very reluctant to break the Oxford arrangement and let down my recommending senior back home, I pulled out. I applied for fellows jobs in both Boston and Adelaide Children's hospitals, gaining the latter position. Although I eventually turned the Adelaide job down explaining my illness as the reason, the senior surgeon there wrote me a threatening letter. He thought I was unprofessional. I felt he was threatening my career. From then on I felt that other colleagues were judging me also.

I wasn't getting the sleep I desperately needed since I woke early each day. I got up feeling exhausted and stressed, then Pamela took me to the rail station in the dark and freezing cold of the Toronto winter. On arrival at the hospital after the 45 minute two-train trip from our rented house in the suburbs, the last thing I felt like doing was face the challenges ahead. Twice on the train home, exhausted, I fell asleep, waking down the line. Pamela had to save my bacon by driving to pick me up. Having a sick husband and alone in suburbia, few friends and often trapped indoors in the harsh winter, she was also stressed. My illness was disrupting the family. It all seemed beyond me. Although lonely and desperate, I told nobody at my work about my distress – I felt ashamed. One morning I could hardly face entering the ward; I had to first clean my face and glasses from the tears of a severe anxiety attack. It was time to admit I needed help.

I consulted a psychiatrist, who first prescribed medication. When I didn't improve he tried hypnosis – also no good as I wouldn't go under. None of the conventional treatments were helping, so as a last effort, he offered me electroconvulsive therapy. This was a controversial treatment, but as a medical student I had been taught that in some cases it could be safe and effective. Pamela was horrified. She was my rock, 'We've got to find somebody else. I won't let you go through with that.'

So I saw another shrink who suited me much better. He suggested, and I agreed to a two week admission to Sunnybrook Hospital.

Sunnybrook was set among green, rolling parkland. Once a private farm, the land had been donated largely for public use and partly for the hospital which now houses the largest trauma centre in Canada. I knew the hospital as I had attended teaching sessions there provided by the orthopaedic surgeons for trainees and fellows like myself. My admission was to the area devoted to treating patients with anxiety and related conditions: trauma to the psyche. The atmosphere was a haven of calm in the ward, and beauty outside. The staff were caring and highly professional. I joined them in group therapy with the other shell-shocked. We shared our stories and distress. Being taken away from the stress of surgery and working on my problems with others, I soon felt better. Since arriving in Toronto, I had done no regular exercise which had been an important part of creating well-being and balance in my life back home. I went on long restorative runs around the sun-lit hospital grounds in the park. Day-by-day I felt stronger, and soon, although still shaky, I was strong enough to get back on the horse.

16.

Arthroscopy

AFTER A YEAR AT TORONTO GENERAL, I moved to Toronto Western Hospital as a resident, the equivalent of a New Zealand registrar. The chief there was another pioneering knee surgeon, Robert Wilson Jackson. I'd heard of Jackson as he had recently published *Arthroscopy of the Knee*, a book he'd co-authored with David Dandy, an English surgeon, but I was not fully aware of his contribution to orthopaedics and disabled athletes.

Jackson had visited Tokyo in 1964 on a travelling scholarship, intending to study tissue culture techniques. While there, he'd helped as a doctor for the Canadian Olympic team, and two weeks later at the Paralympics.

His disappointment that Canada did not have a team at the Paralympics spurred him into action. He became one of the founding fathers of the Canadian Paralympic Movement and the Canadian Wheelchair Sport Association.

While in Tokyo, he tracked down a surgeon he had heard was practising a new technique – 'arthroscopy'. (The term was first used by a Danish surgeon, Severin Nordentoft, who in 1912 wrote about his use of a primitive endoscope to look into the bladder, abdominal cavity and knee joint.)

Jackson didn't have an easy time finding the surgeon as the technique was not well known, even in Tokyo. The man's name was Masaki Watanabe and he was building on early work by an earlier surgeon, Kenji Tagaki.

Tagaki's earliest experiments had used a small-gauge cystoscope, an instrument for viewing the inside of children's bladders. Through small incisions in the front of the knee, he inserted the cystoscope into the knee joint cavity. He went on to develop 12 iterations, improving the design as he went. Watanabe followed him, eventually replacing the earlier incandescent light source with much improved fibre ('cold') light technology in his 21st model.

Watanabe taught Jackson arthroscopy in two sessions per week over several months, in return for Jackson helping his Japanese tutor learn English. Jackson then brought the technique back to Canada. He encountered scepticism. In an article for the *Journal of Arthroscopy* in October 2009, he quoted a prominent US orthopaedic surgeon saying, 'Why look through the keyhole when you can open the door?' Another surgeon called it an 'instrument of the devil'.

John Goodfellow, who would co-develop the Oxford knee replacement, referred to the arthroscope as the 'illuminated knee gouge'. The remark was tongue-in-cheek, but it does point to the fact that inexperienced surgeons (and even well-practised ones) could unintentionally scrape the smooth surface of the cartilage while manoeuvring the instrument in the narrow spaces of the knee. Those of us who started learning the technique were practising on our patients. This was not ideal: cartilage injuries heal poorly.

There were other teething problems. The optical and electrical components of the arthroscope could not withstand high heat. On several occasions the instrument was inadvertently heat-sterilised by nurses and had to be sent back to Japan for repair.

Despite these setbacks Jackson persisted. According to an editorial in the *Journal of Arthroscopy* in January 2010, he noted that he was able to teach it only one-on-one. 'There were no visual aids, no videos, nothing.'

I would find the same thing when I returned to New Zealand. Crouching over the operating table using one eye to view the inside of a knee through the scope, I was the only person in the room who knew what was happening.

This made it difficult both to properly learn and then teach arthroscopic techniques. This was just as well. I was painfully slow to gain the necessary skills and quite pleased others couldn't see my clumsy early operations.

In time, instructional courses began using plastic models, human cadavers and pigs' joints for practice. It was not until the early 1980s, when modern optics and video became available, that the procedure was transformed: I could stand in comfort and others in theatre could share the view.

When I worked with Jackson, arthroscopy was still in its infancy. Using a camera and an arthroscope, or 'joint' telescope, surgeons were learning to guide fine instruments through small stab incisions – a process known as keyhole surgery – rather than the previous large open incisions. These small incisions greatly reduced post-operative pain and so sped up recovery. Whereas an 'open' operation might have required several days of pain relief in a hospital, with keyhole surgery the patient could be in and out in a day.

Many of his Jackson's patients were sportspeople. They knew that if their knee injury was treated with conventional surgery a lengthy recovery might follow. For professionals, the surgery might even end their career. When they saw that keyhole surgery was leading to fast recovery, they quickly caught on. Newspaper articles about top athletes whose rapid recovery was due to the method helped spread

Arthroscopy

the word. Arthroscopy surgeons became in high demand.

In 1968, with his pupils and other surgeons, Jackson formed the International Arthroscopy Association at a conference of the American Academy of Orthopaedic Surgeons in Las Vegas. Masaki Watanabe was elected president, and Jackson vice president. Intrigue surrounded the association's early days. In 1970, at a course in arthroscopy in Philadelphia, a meeting was held in a hotel room. President Richard Nixon, visiting the city, was staying in the same hotel so the meeting took place under the intense surveillance of secret service agents, suspicious about what the group of young men gathered in a room in the same hotel were up to. They locked the surgeons in the room for around four hours until the president departed.

In 1975 the association's first formal meeting was held in Copenhagen. Eight founding members had each paid a sub of US$500. Richard O'Connor, the first treasurer, had converted the $4000 into gold coins, mostly South African Krugerrands, despite there being a moratorium in the United States on the private ownership of gold. O'Connor carried the coins in a money belt around his waist on the flight to Copenhagen. After the meeting he went to Switzerland, opened a numbered bank account and deposited them. In 1977 the association's officeholders elected to sell the gold. The amount realised was approximately $60,000, a profit of $56,000 after only two years.

Jackson's work with athletes and the disabled gained him recognition and awards. In 1994 *Sports Illustrated* named him as one of the 40 individuals (and the only physician) who'd had the most significant impact on sports in the previous 40 years. When he died in 2010, his eulogy acknowledged that his 'modest and soft-spoken demeanour belied the magnitude of his accomplishments and contributions … [which were] nothing short of revolutionising surgery as it is practised across almost all fields.' His promotion of arthroscopy helped spread keyhole surgery throughout the world, not only for orthopaedic conditions: today endoscopes are routinely used to perform minimally invasive surgery throughout the body.

While I was working with Jackson, we were living in downtown Toronto where Pamela had the support of neighbours in our multi-storey university apartment block. She was enjoying the stimulus; it was a major relief after suburban isolation. Our children were settled and attending a local school. But I was struggling. I was again experiencing depressive episodes. I felt tense and low in confidence. The work routine was still too hard and I had neither time nor energy to exercise enough or engage in interests outside my job – I was either at work or home exhausted. I also felt a failure as a husband and father, not being able to help Pamela with the children. Although

Arthroscopy

Pamela was not pleased to leave, we decided to cut short our Canadian stay.

On the plane heading back to New Zealand, I brightened up as I talked rugby with a fellow Kiwi. I had played one game in Toronto. A doctor at the hospital had heard I was a New Zealander and had played rugby. Thinking we Kiwis could all perform like All Blacks, he bludgeoned me into the hospital social team. We played on a hot summer day. I hadn't done much physical activity for months. At the end of the game, I lay on the ground exhausted and dehydrated, trying to recover enough energy to grasp a cold beer. But then came a nasty surprise. Instead of slaking their thirst, the team sat around and smoked dope.

17.

Some Doctors Eat Their Young

AFTER I RETURNED FROM TORONTO, having had a break and mainly recovered from my crippling depression I needed a job. I rang the professor of orthopaedics in Auckland to arrange a discussion about my job prospects at Middlemore. When I arrived for the interview, I was surprised to find the boss there: this had not been discussed. I feared my previous relationship with him would count against me. It did. The interview was short. I told them of the stress I had experienced in Toronto and the factors that had precipitated it. I said that after treatment and back in a familiar environment, I felt able to start up again. I told them I had gained major new skills in knee surgery and innovative Swiss fracture fixation techniques.

They were unsympathetic. There seemed to be no interest in the skills I'd acquired. They clearly saw me as weak, and unsuitable for a job in Auckland. I remembered the old adage: 'Some doctors eat their young.' I was in the presence of medico-cannibals. They showed me the door.

I was shaken and upset. I could see why they might be cautious, but they had seemed unnecessarily harsh.

There was to be a corollary a few years later. After becoming established as an orthopaedic surgeon in Wellington, I began getting referrals from around the country, particularly from injured athletes. A few came from Auckland. At a conference in Wellington, an Auckland surgeon sidled up to me. 'The boss has been told that you are accepting patients from Auckland. He wants you to stop this.'

I was incredulous. The boss had summarily turned me away from Auckland and showed no interest in the skills I had brought back from Toronto. Now he wanted me to stop using these skills to help patients. I responded quietly but firmly, 'With all respect to you and the boss, I accept patients who seek my help from anywhere in the country and will continue to do so. I would be grateful if you could pass that on.' I heard no more.

After my trauma in Toronto and rejection in Auckland, my interest in returning to the cut and thrust of orthopaedics waned. I needed time out. I doubted anyone would employ me anyway: the small New Zealand orthopaedic bush telegraph works well. My previous experience in general practice had taught me that I could be competent and happy in a locum job if I didn't have to do obstetrics. I had also learnt that I liked working in rural areas, where I could enjoy the outdoors.

An ideal opportunity came up in Queenstown. The Central Otago town was relatively quiet, not the bustling tourist mecca it has since become. An added attraction was that Pamela's parents had recently retired to nearby Arrowtown. Before we left Toronto, we had been living in the inner city, where Pamela had made friends with women with children of a similar age to ours. It had been a major wrench to leave this comfortable environment and return to New Zealand. I hoped a move to Queenstown might act as some compensation.

I hadn't been there long when I got an urgent call. 'Can you get out to the airport urgently to meet Don Spary. He'll chopper you into Skippers Canyon. A motorcyclist has gone over a bluff.'

My heart raced as we took off into the air. Within minutes we saw the young man. He was lying motionless beside his motorbike, about 20 metres below the notorious Skippers Road and high above a deep gorge.

Spary was celebrated for his helicopter handling skills.

Some Doctors Eat Their Young

I now saw why. The slope was far from ideal – steep-sided with a constant danger of the rotor blades hitting a side of the cliff – but he landed gently on a flattish area about 20 metres from the man.

I managed to crab my way along the rock face carrying a stretcher. The man, who looked to be in his late teens, was unresponsive. I couldn't see or feel any buckled limbs, but there was a nasty abrasion on his head. He was breathing and had a pulse, but it was very weak. He was deeply unconscious but alive.

With difficulty, I strapped him onto the stretcher. Hovering over me in the helicopter, Spary let down a rope. I grabbed it and somehow pushed the young man and the stretcher into the chopper before clambering in myself. 'Watch out,' Spary yelled as we roared into the air. 'Bloody hell, you nearly put us into the cliff,' he added.

As we flew back to the airport it took all my strength to hold on to the stretcher, with the patient's lower legs and feet hanging in thin air outside the cramped cabin. Back in the resuscitation area of the small Queenstown hospital, I assessed the patient's condition. He had a bad head injury and possibly a broken neck. There was no time to waste. I put him in a neck collar and loaded him into an ambulance for a fast trip to Invercargill Hospital. I learnt next day that he had died overnight.

A month later, I left general practice forever.

Anxious to return to orthopaedics. I started to look around for jobs outside Auckland. I went to a job interview in Rotorua. The head of department was Māori. He asked me whether I was familiar with Māori culture. 'You will have to treat many with a Māori background here.'

I told him I didn't speak te reo but had trained among the Māori community in South Auckland at Middlemore Hospital. I had treated many Māori children, particularly in the club foot clinic. I had also worked alongside Māori in holiday jobs as a student and was sympathetic to Māori aspirations. Apparently, this was not enough: he shooed me away.

I visited the professor of orthopaedics at Dunedin Hospital. When the prof had lectured us at medical school, he had come across as a rigid and testy character but an entertaining teacher. I still remember some of his idiosyncratic messages. Referring to X-ray images of bones that had died through lack of blood, he would bombastically proclaim, 'Dead bone is white bone, white bone is dead bone.'

After showing us an X-ray of a simple forearm fracture, he'd asked a member of the class, 'How are you going to treat this?'

Silence.

'Well,' he demanded, 'what are you going to do? Kiss it? Rub water on it? Sprinkle it with hundreds and thousands?'

Some Doctors Eat Their Young

On another occasion he asked one of my classmates, 'You there, can you tell me the clinical signs and initial treatment for a patient who has fallen on his outstretched hand? The X-ray of the wrist is negative and you have diagnosed a possible fractured scaphoid.'

The scaphoid is a key bone, one of eight in the wrist. When fractured, it is prone to either fail to heal or, worse, partially die because of disturbance to its blood supply. Eventually osteoarthritis of the wrist may develop, so the injury must be treated early and well. The diagnosis of a broken scaphoid bone is occasionally missed as the black fracture line in the white bone may not be apparent on initial X-rays. The recommended practice is to treat the wrist as if there is a fracture, then X-ray it about two weeks after the injury. By then, the line is usually visible if the bone is broken.

My classmate was speechless. The prof: 'Anybody?' More speechlessness. 'Well,' he said, 'if you're not going to learn the basics of fracture management, I'm not going to waste my time on you.' With that he strode regally out of the class, never to return.

I had a small personal connection with the prof. When I was a child, he had treated my father for a rupture of his patellar tendon, the thick 'rope' that anchors the kneecap to the main lower leg bone. My father had attempted to throw a heavy metal ball in a shot-put contest at a school reunion. He'd slipped on the grass and the point of his knee had struck a stake in the ground. His kneecap had been pushed up into his lower thigh, far north of its rightful position. The doctor's job had been to put it back in place. My father had been off work for a long time, but the repair had been successful. He thought the prof a 'really good bloke'.

He was a prominent member of the New Zealand Orthopaedic Association and winner of many academic prizes. A major achievement was his role in setting up the national orthopaedic registrar training scheme, of which he was the first chair. His obituary would describe him as 'a gifted and witty university medical teacher'. But he could also be cruel.

His insults to female medical students were legendary. Also to female nurses. One involved an incident in an operating theatre. The female scrub nurse had handed him an instrument he didn't like. 'What's wrong with you?' he said to her. 'Got the rags on?'

Female radiographers were fair game. They regularly left his operating room in tears after being insulted. Race, religion and body shape were other targets for ridicule. A colleague remembered his comment when an injured Pacific Island man was being used in class as a case study. 'Now, tell us what happened to you. You fell out of a coconut tree?'

He constantly addressed a male student who had a gently curving nose and a black beard as 'rabbi'. He disapproved of medical students who wore their hair long. Of one hirsute classmate he said, 'I see we have Jesus among us.' The man was then grilled mercilessly on his knowledge of orthopaedic topics. In an operation where the patient was an overweight woman, the prof lifted an apron of fat and skin: 'A thing of beauty is a joy forever. The human form comes in a multitude of manifestations.'

Understandably, I was nervous when I met him for an interview at his holiday home, about nine months after returning from Toronto. I could see another lion's den experience coming up.

He sat me down in his garden. 'What orthopaedics did you do in Toronto?'

'As a fellow I covered general orthopaedics,' I said, 'including acute injuries. I was keen to learn the new Swiss fixation methods for fractures and joined the orthopaedic trainees.'

I added, 'I worked with two great knee surgeons. You'll know Bob Jackson and David MacIntosh?'

He grunted. 'What academic activities?' I replied that I had carried out research on MacIntosh's ACL reconstruction patients and presented some results at an annual scientific meeting of the Canadian Orthopaedic Association.

He interrupted. 'Well,' he said, 'we don't have a position for you. If we did have, you'd have to keep your nose clean.' He seemed to equate my stress-related illness to a nasal infection. He didn't have a door in his garden, but he metaphorically showed me one.

Later he invited me to speak on ACL tears, their clinical signs and treatment methods, at an orthopaedic conference he organised in Dunedin. Not long after I spoke, he wrote to me. 'Dear Mr Tregonning. I have just seen a patient of yours in my clinic. You had performed an ACL reconstruction. I just want to tell you that your operation has failed.'

I was perplexed. What did he mean by 'failed'? I valued feedback from surgeons who saw my patients elsewhere after my surgery, but this brief note seemed a deliberate attempt to discourage me. I was given no details, nor asked to get further involved in the case. This was strange. Looking back, the incident smacks of a man in power asserting his dominance. He didn't want me to think I could walk on water. At the time I was angry at the putdown, but in retrospect I should have taken steps to find out more and ensure the patient was all right.

The orthopaedic community in New Zealand is small. The consultants on whom I was reliant for an appointment to a permanent position knew my history. Most had little knowledge of anxiety and clinical depression, nor how common these conditions were (and still are) among junior doctors.

Today, stress-induced conditions are better known

and talked about. When I became president of the New Zealand Orthopaedic Association I chose, as my initiative, to foster a surgeon support service along the lines of the one operated by the Australian association. The service has since been replaced by a pan-surgical support service run by the Royal Australasian College of Surgeons. Its website notes: 'Surgeons, like the rest of society, can struggle with depression, anxiety and poor mental health. The work environments surgeons find themselves in may also contribute to high levels of stress due to administrative processes, fear of litigation and inappropriate behaviour such as bullying, discrimination and sexual harassment.'

Bullying is now actively discouraged: 'The College will encourage work and training environments free of bullying, sexual harassment and unlawful discrimination. It should be understood that these unreasonable behaviours will not be tolerated under any circumstances.'

In 1978, my dream of an enhanced career with the Toronto experience under my belt was shattered. Fortunately, this was only temporary. I was down, but not out.

18.

Knees Up

In August I joined Tauranga Hospital as a senior orthopaedic registrar. I was glad to be back in Tauranga and again working in orthopaedics. I started performing the MacIntosh reconstruction operations I had learnt in Toronto, but arthroscopy had to wait: there was no arthroscope in the hospital.

After three months, Bill Gillespie recommended I take up a job at Wellington Hospital. In Toronto I had happily joined the tie-less brigade after wearing a tie and jacket for 13 years. When I joined Wellington Hospital, I was taken aside by my immediate senior. 'The head of department wants you to wear a tie.' That night I considered my options. I was 33, but still relatively junior in the orthopaedic pecking order. I couldn't afford to rock the boat. For the next 30 years I wore what I regarded as an antiquated and completely pointless status symbol.

After two years I was appointed a full-time surgeon. Most of my elective surgery and clinics were at Kenepuru Hospital in Porirua, 23 kilometres north of my home in Karori. I also performed acute-roster weekend duties and regular clinics at Hutt Hospital, 20 kilometres in another direction, and began some private work. Initially most of this was at the Wellington Surgical Clinic in the CBD, the first day-care surgical hospital in Australasia. Soon I began in-patient private surgery at Bowen Hospital in the northern suburbs. As I drove around Wellington between these hospitals, I listened to and sang taped music. I had joined the Orpheus Choir and found the car a perfect place to learn the bass part of the choral repertoire.

I was disappointed that most of my senior colleagues seemed to have little interest in the new and transformative knee concepts and techniques I had learnt in Toronto. In 1980 I offered a paper to the *New Zealand Medical Journal* on the diagnosis of knee ligament injuries. It was rejected. I was told I had overemphasised the importance of injuries to the anterior cruciate ligament. I had to revise the paper to have it accepted, although my main message remained the same.

Blood and Bone

The medical establishment is inherently conservative. Changes take time to be accepted. This scepticism about new procedures is a good thing. New operations need testing; they should show better results than existing techniques or no surgery and the results need to be repeated. My paper described concepts that were not known well in New Zealand. I was a relative unknown, wet behind the ears and a bit breathless, just back from overseas. I was possibly seen as a know-all young upstart and a bit dodgy.

I carefully kept data on all my knee patients and wrote papers for *New Zealand Medical Journal*, *New Zealand Journal of Sports Medicine* and a nursing publication, *The Dissector*. Bill, keen to encourage his colleagues to specialise, encouraged me to set up a knee injuries clinic at Wellington Hospital; at the time it was the only specialised knee clinic in the country.

I lectured on knee injuries to doctors, nurses, physiotherapists and sportspeople. Newspapers began to run stories on my work, so when I started private practice word got out. People with ACL injuries that had caused them years of disabling instability made appointments. Injured athletes who wanted a quick recovery and return to sport lined up for knee arthroscopy. Without ever intending it, I was now a knee specialist. People I worked with started to call me 'the knee man'.

Trying to persuade nurses to allow patients to go

home on the day of their knee arthroscopy was a struggle at first. The protocol was to allow patients to be discharged after surgery only if they had passed urine. Closed surgery patients had been starved for at least four hours before surgery so they had empty bladders. Eventually the requirement to urinate was dropped; most patients limped out as soon as they'd recovered from the anaesthetic.

Keith, aged 65, recently told me his story. 'When I was a university student in 1978, I twisted my right knee badly and had continuing pain,' he said. 'At Wellington Hospital the surgeon did a meniscectomy in the old way. It was very painful afterwards. I was kept in hospital for several days, then attended physiotherapy for several weeks.

'In 2000 I was dancing up a storm when I caught my other foot on the floor. More pain and instability, this time in my left knee. You said to me, "I reckon you'll be back biking in six weeks." The day after you operated, my son got injured and I drove him to A&E no problem. I had no physiotherapy and was back on my mountain bike within six weeks. The difference was night and day.'

My close colleague in innovative knee surgery, Barry Tietjens, spearheaded the formation of the New Zealand Knee Society and proposed me as the first president. Barry and I had worked together at Auckland Hospital in the early '70s. We had both gained our early interest in knee surgery with John Cullen. Barry had furthered that interest at Oxford University, and after returning to New Zealand had organised knee arthroscopy training courses for New Zealand surgeons.

The society had its inaugural meeting at Okawa Bay near Rotorua in 1992. It has since morphed into the New Zealand Knee and Sports Surgery Society and meets annually, with visiting overseas speakers and presentations from local researchers.

In 1983 I had a paper published in the British *Journal of Bone and Joint Surgery* in which I reported on a series of my patients with unstable meniscus tears who had complained of painful 'mechanical symptoms' – jamming, clicking or clunking, or true 'locking'. In a previous paper in the *New Zealand Medical Journal* I'd compared closed and open surgery for common meniscal tears. Both papers reported on how long it took patients to return to work: two and a half times longer after an open operation than a closed one. I concluded that patients would benefit if the closed surgery were used more widely. Furthermore, there would be economic benefits. Meniscectomy was the country's most common elective orthopaedic operation with up to 2,500 performed each year, predominantly on young men of working age.

Conclusions made by operating surgeons researching their own patients' results are considered weaker than those of independent researchers because of perceived bias.

Knees Up

When I later became an editor for the *Journal of Bone and Joint Surgery*, I always took this into account when assessing papers for publication. But the new techniques I described were clearly considered important. My papers sneaked past the reviewers.

Today, closed methods are the accepted method of treating meniscal injuries that are causing certain 'mechanical' symptoms. The technique mostly gives patients a relatively pain-free experience with a quick recovery and little risk of complications. But a problem has arisen: some surgeons arthroscope knees too often, particularly in middle-aged and elderly patients with osteoarthritis.

I was recently reminded of this when I met a man named Jack. He looked vaguely familiar. He asked for my name. When I told him, he immediately asked what I did. I'm usually cautious about telling people my job. All too often I get the familiar response: 'Oh, you'll be fascinated by this.' The person will then regale me with a long-winded tale of an operation they/their wife/mother/child/cousin or some distant relative has had. I'm seldom fascinated.

Jack said, 'Oh, I'm about to have a knee replacement with one of your colleagues. He's already done four arthroscopies on my knee.'

'Oh, so you've had further injuries to the knee?'

'No,' Jack said, 'it's just got more worn and painful.'

Oh, I thought, so we're still doing it.

To some people, orthopaedics and a limp go together. There is an old joke: 'If you go into a town and don't see anyone limping, you know that no orthopaedic surgeon works there.' Pamela and I were in Queenstown one day on holiday. Walking down the street we noticed a man limping badly. I whispered to Pamela, 'Gee, that man needs to see an orthopod.' We drew up alongside him. 'Crikey,' I whispered, 'he's one of mine. Quick, let's duck into this side street.'

The unfortunate man hobbled into the distance. Down the road, we entered a shop. Turning into an aisle I met my old patient face-to-face. Embarrassed, I blurted out, 'Oh, hello. How's your knee?'

'No good,' he muttered. 'Still bloody sore, I'm off to see another surgeon.'

The job as an orthopaedic surgeon brings much satisfaction, but when things go wrong I rank it up there among the worst.

Arthroscopy and closed surgery were the highlights of my early career. My next breakthrough came through others introducing me to a less invasive form of knee-replacement surgery: the Oxford 'uni'. The uni, short for unicompartmental, replaces only one compartment of the knee joint, most often the inside (medial). Like most other orthopaedic surgeons I was most often replacing both main compartments of osteoarthritic knees with conventional fixed-bearing total knee replacements, and occasionally uni or half replacements, through large incisions. In the mid-1980s I visited both sides of the Atlantic to learn from two innovators. At Nuffield Orthopaedic Centre in Oxford I visited John Goodfellow, the developer of the Oxford prosthesis. Unfortunately, no Oxford uni knee operation was being done while I was there, but John generously sat me down and asked, 'What do you need to know?' He then explained the technique at length.

I was interested but not convinced. There were reports in the literature of the mobile bearing dislocating.

I next visited John Insall, an Englishman who worked at the Hospital for Special Surgery in New York. Insall, a superb surgeon and teacher, had worked with an engineer, Albert Burstein, to develop a knee prosthesis. Its unique features were the shaping of the bearing surfaces to better reduce wear of the plastic and metal. The posterior cruciate ligament was replaced with a plastic peg to ensure stability. Insall also emphasised the importance of manipulating ligaments on the side of the knee to prevent deformity – the most common known as bow leg.

In 1998, the Oxford group altered the design of its prosthesis and the instrumentation, so it could be implanted via a small incision. This incision was only about half the size of the one we were using. I quickly learnt the technique. Because I had narrowed my practice solely to knee surgery, I gained experience fast. Patients were, in the main, pleased. I presented my results at conferences and lectured on the subject. I also assisted at 'saw-bones' sessions, helping teach other surgeons insertion using dummy plastic knees.

In 2006, I was invited with two other New Zealanders to an international conference at Blenheim Palace to celebrate the 30-year anniversary of the Oxford uni, as it had become known. I presented New Zealand's experience with all unis, including the Oxford, giving a comparative analysis of the results using data from the New Zealand Joint Registry. My five-minute paper was the last of 42 and took place at the end of the second day. John Goodfellow was in the front row. I occasionally squinted to see if he was asleep or looked bored. He looked neither but may have been a good actor.

I admired Insall and Goodfellow, but this was not my main reason for using their prostheses. It was the results, as shown in the international registries and in my own patients.

In 2010 I visited the US again as a senior member of the Asia Pacific Orthopaedic Society for Sports Medicine. My role was to guide three younger travelling fellows from the Asia Pacific during visits to eight cities. At each centre we presented papers. From experience, I had come to realise that many older patients gained no benefit from arthroscopic surgery. A very controversial paper about this had appeared in the *New England Journal of Medicine*. A group of US surgeons had compared real with sham arthroscopic knee surgery on patients with osteoarthritis of the knee. Sham surgery is a fake operation where the part of the surgery thought to be beneficial is omitted. The sham acts as a control: its results are compared with those of the real operation, just like a placebo in drug research trials. The patients did not know the type of surgery they would receive; they had consented to the fact they might get the sham procedure.

The sham operations had been performed with the patients sedated but awake. The surgeon, hidden from the patient, called for scalpel, arthroscope and instruments as he would for the real arthroscopy, but put no instruments into the knee joint. Two small skin incisions were made, then sewn up identical in size and position to those on patients who received the real procedures. The results had shown no significant difference in the outcome.

Some prominent American arthroscopy surgeons had been highly defensive and sceptical about the results of the study. At Ann Arbor in Michigan I presented a literature review on the topic to an orthopaedic audience, arguing that we shouldn't be arthroscoping worn knees unless there was a clear injury and a definitely torn and treatable structure. I expected robust discussion. There was none. Maybe the surgeons agreed with me? Or maybe they disagreed but were too polite to challenge me? I was disappointed: I was looking forward to hearing their views.

Patients with osteoarthritic knees can often get relief from non-surgical treatments such as regular exercise, physiotherapy, perhaps anti-inflammatory pills or a steroid injection. I had come to realise it was wise to try all non-surgical treatments before considering surgery.

Tears of the meniscus in the uninjured knee of an older person are common. Studies using magnetic resonance imaging – MRI – show that more than half of elderly people have meniscal tears without symptoms. This is because as the body ages the menisci become weakened by normal wear and tear. Where there are pain and other symptoms it's mainly because of worn cartilage. Cartilage has no feeling. However, when it's thin, flaking and even worn completely away it exposes the underlying bone, which is pain sensitive. The rough cartilage – or, even worse, the bone grinding on bone – increases friction in the joint and may cause symptoms such as sticking, catching or temporary locking.

Inflammation is caused by particles coming off the deteriorating joint surfaces. These annoy the lining of the knee; it becomes swollen and produces a fluid that makes the joint swell. Arthroscopy allows vision inside the knee if the joint is irrigated with saline solution. This continuous flow washes out the particles and can therefore reduce inflammation and relieve pain.

The procedure may bring short-lived relief. The surgeon may think the improvement is due to the surgery. In fact, studies have shown that simply irrigating the knee with saline solution can have as much effect as partial removal of the torn meniscus fragment and 'cleaning up' the joint surface by removing loose cartilage, a process known as debridement. Arthroscopic procedures in older patients are not harmless. Research has shown an accelerated need for knee replacement compared to patients who haven't had interventions.

Arthroscopic knee surgeries are still regularly performed; they are among the most common private orthopaedic operations. They are a nice little earner that can benefit surgeons more than patients.

A knee problem that *is* helped by arthroscopy is a 'joint mouse'. Composed of bone with a layer of cartilage, mice may be formed by broken-off growths at the edge of arthritic joints. They are small (often about the size of a fingernail) and so can move around within the large joint space and hide in the narrow tunnel-like extensions. A mouse may jump out of its hole and get caught between the moving parts of the joint, causing the knee to lock. It is easily removed arthroscopically.

In some patients a mouse is a fragment of dead bone caused by blood supply near the surface of a joint being disturbed. The fragment (with overlying cartilage) can loosen and fall into the knee joint cavity. This condition is called osteochondritis dissecans – the fragment 'dissects' itself from healthy bone. It occurs most often in children and adolescents, especially those involved in high-impact activities such as jumping and running. It can affect not only the knee but elbows, ankles and other joints. In young children it can heal by itself: doctors advise stopping vigorous activities to encourage this.

John was an active 15-year-old when his father brought him to see me. 'I haven't had an injury but my knee hurts and catches at times when I twist, particularly playing football,' John told me. 'It feels as if it might jam up but doesn't completely. I think it swells a bit. I've had to give all my sport away.'

I examined John's knee and showed him and his father the X-ray on my screen. 'See this separated bit of bone,' I said. 'It's whiter than the rest. That means it's dead and floating about. I'll probably have to fix it back in place with pins or screws.' I answered their questions and booked John for surgery.

At arthroscopy a probe showed a piece of cartilage and

Knees Up

a fragment of underlying dead bone were mostly detached. I could pull the nearly completely loose piece into the joint. I had to try and get a blood supply to the fragment when I manipulated it back into place. I made a skin incision of a few centimetres to gain access to the joint and scraped scar tissue off the bone, leaving a hole. I harvested some live bone from just outside the joint and filled the hole. After putting the loose piece snugly back I screwed it firmly in place. The cartilage of the fixed fragment surface was now flush with its surrounds.

I shared the triumph with the theatre staff. 'Look what we have done, team. That piece is back rock-solid. Is that perfect or what?' I was stoked.

John's knee healed, and after a second minor operation to remove the screws he went on to play sport again. We had killed a mouse just before its birth.

19.

Scope for Surgery

KENEPURU HOSPITAL WAS BUILT IN THE late 1970s in the grounds of Porirua Psychiatric Hospital, which had started life in 1887 as the Porirua Lunatic Asylum. At one time, Porirua was the largest hospital in New Zealand; about 20 kilometres of roads criss-crossed its 42-hectare grounds. Patients ranged from people with mental illness to the senile and alcoholic.

Just before I arrived in Wellington the first psychiatric ward had closed and from the late 1980s, while I worked at adjacent Kenepuru, Porirua Hospital patients were progressively released into the community and many of the buildings removed. In 2014, land around the hospital was bought by the local iwi, Ngāti Toa, and as I write a huge housing complex is being built on it.

I held a weekly fracture clinic at Kenepuru. Recently clerk Hine Simpson and I reminisced about our experiences at Kenepuru in the old days. Hine told me she came to work at Kenepuru from a job at Porirua Hospital as a seamstress in the late 1970s.

My interest was aroused. 'What were you sewing?'

'Straitjackets,' she said.

I knew these had been used way back when but had thought they'd disappeared. We'd been taught at medical school that they'd been replaced by tranquillisers and anti-depressant drugs (the medical straightjackets).

Hine said ECT (electroconvulsive treatment) was common in the back room of the ward. By then people undergoing the treatment were given muscle relaxants and sedatives. Without these drugs, ECT had occasionally caused orthopaedic problems. A rare but serious complication was fracture or dislocation of the long bones of the arms and legs caused by the violent muscular contractions during the medically induced convulsion.

Kenepuru's operating theatres were underused when I started operating there in 1981. Hospital management encouraged me to do as much operating as I could. For a young surgeon like me this was a dream come true. All junior surgeons want to get as much cutting as possible to develop their craft. Wellington Hospital was a hotbed of hospital politics, with constant struggles between specialties to get enough operating time in the theatres. By comparison Kenepuru was nearly politics-free. I loved the freedom. I could arthroscope any injured knee that wouldn't move. I could operate as much as I wanted.

My enthusiasm for arthroscopy was not shared by everyone. In a paper published in the *New Zealand Medical Journal*, I reviewed the results of my first 200 diagnostic arthroscopy patients. This prompted an Auckland radiologist to comment in a letter to the editor: 'Tregonning gives a pre-eminence to arthroscopy unsupported by the evidence.' He didn't quote the evidence. The alternative, arthrography, involved injecting liquid into the knee by a radiologist, where it showed up white on an X-ray film. With injuries of the meniscus, the liquid would hopefully seep into a tear in the cartilage but in cases I saw, it didn't always do so; I greatly preferred arthroscopy. Today, arthroscopy is still alive. Knee arthrography has died a natural death.

In recent years MRI has replaced arthroscopy for diagnosing knee conditions: it shows soft tissues and bone in superb detail, is cheaper than arthroscopy and non-invasive. Cutting into a joint, even via small stab wounds, can cause infection, nerve damage, pain or increased sensitivity when kneeling, and deep vein thrombosis. On rare occasions a clot will get to the lung. This is potentially fatal.

Scope for Surgery

Such serious events are very unusual.

But there are also problems with MRI. It can show there is a meniscal tear, but not if the piece torn is loose enough to catch and cause pain. At worst, diagnosis of a meniscal tear may encourage unnecessary surgery.

Initially, I had a very limited array of arthroscopic instruments. Few had been developed and were available commercially. I experimented with other surgeons' tools and broke several ear, nose and throat instruments. There was a lot of swearing. I became expert at retrieving bust-off bits of metal from inside my patients' knees.

One of my favourite instruments was pituitary forceps. This was designed for surgery on the pituitary gland in the brain. Its smooth rounded profile and angled sharp cutting edge allowed me to do hundreds of operations without harming delicate cartilage before instruments designed especially for the job became available.

I was sometimes handed blunt or otherwise unsatisfactory instruments for other types of open operations. 'This bloody thing is completely unsuitable,' I remember saying. 'Haven't we got something sharper?' And 'I've got tools in my workshop that beat this hands down.' And 'Back home, I'd toss this thing in the bin.' I had been conditioned by my carpenter father, who kept his tools in immaculate condition.

Blood and Bone

I sometimes couldn't find better tools in the theatre inventory, or get the existing ones rehabilitated. Fighting to get new gear was always a hassle. Either it was not available or it was considered too expensive. More than once I bought a sharp tool at a hardware shop and put it through the autoclave to sterilise it. I never told the hospital hierarchy about my innovations. No patient suffered. My frame of mind benefitted.

There is a popular misconception among the public that it takes unusual manual skills to become a surgeon. In fact, I have only average manual skills, some learnt in my father's workshop. He taught me how to hold and use tools, instructions I found useful in theatre. 'When you use a saw, Russ, always point your index finger down the saw blade,' he said more than once. 'Don't push or pull down hard. Just let the teeth do the work.'

Sawing through a tibia during a below-knee amputation, or less often through a femur, I would remember his advice: Let the saw do the work. I disliked these operations intensely; repeating my father's advice like a mantra helped me get through them. Saw, do the work. It wasn't me who was doing this ghastly operation, cutting through the bone and tossing the limb aside, my index finger pointed determinedly downwards. It was the saw.

Despite the best efforts of my father and the woodwork teachers at my Dunedin primary school, I am not a

Scope for Surgery

good carpenter. For a time, Pamela and I owned a small holiday house in Wanaka. A door developed a nasty way of sticking and not closing properly. 'No problem,' I said to Pamela, 'I'll have this fixed in a jiff. I've seen Dad pack up one of the hinges to correct the slope.'

After taking off the door and packing the hinge numerous times, the thing was worse than before. I threw down the tools and went fly-fishing. Meanwhile, Pamela got a real carpenter over. He took one look at the sad hinge work and asked, 'Who did this?' When Pamela said it was her husband, he said, 'Crikey! What on earth does he do for a job?'

I've been told the difference between a violin maestro and an average orchestral player is practice, practice and more practice. Winston Churchill said, 'Continuous effort – not strength or intelligence – is the key to unlocking our potential.' What was required for me to become a surgeon was practice, persistence and patience. It took me years to learn arthroscopic surgery. I could see I would gain great satisfaction and my patients' approval and praise if I could master it, so I kept on.

I knew that if the tourniquet was inflated for too long it might damage the limb due to lack of blood, so I made a rule: if I couldn't finish an operation using the scope within an hour, I would enlarge the incision and perform the surgery in the conventional way.

I must have frustrated many nursing and anaesthetic colleagues with my slow, dogged operating style, but I've comforted myself with the thought that in over 40 years not one patient said, 'Dr Tregonning, I want you to operate on me as fast as you can.'

At Kenepuru I worked with a wide variety of people from all walks of life. Many worked at nearby Todd Motors, the city's largest car assembly plant, and a large number were Māori or Pasifika. I enjoyed working with them and liked the close-knit environment. Smaller hospitals have fewer workers, less bureaucracy, and less dead space in the buildings, with short corridors making for quick movements for staff and patients. I appreciated the fast delivery of patients between ward and operating theatre, a boon for getting my operating list finished before the end of the day.

At Wellington Hospital, I occasionally rushed up to a ward to wheel my next patient to theatre when no orderly was available. This was not a problem at Kenepuru: we treated few acutely injured patients and so there was less pressure on theatre time and staff. The downside was that the theatres were chronically underused; theatre nursing staff would be directed to work at Wellington Hospital when there were no operations scheduled because of the lack of a surgeon or anaesthetist.

In acute hospitals such as Wellington, patients for

elective surgery are often bumped off the list. I was distressed when my patients had starved and steeled themselves for surgery, taken time off work and possibly made family arrangements, only to be told at the last minute to go home. Occasionally, management or senior nursing staff would ask me to tell patients why they'd been cancelled. 'No, that's not my job,' I'd protest. 'It's not my decision; I'm prepared to stay on and operate. Please get one of the managers to go and explain the situation.'

I agreed with nursing colleagues that it would be unfair to expect them to stay on at the end of their shift, but I thought more could have been done to increase staffing of the theatres and prevent patients who'd already been admitted being booted out the door. I never succeeded with my argument, but unwisely I kept on making it.

I also made representations to the management at Wellington to make more use of Kenepuru for elective surgery. When I visited colleagues in the UK I saw peripheral hospitals used in this way. To get more elective surgery happening, I liaised with a sympathetic manager and two excellent colleagues – a charge nurse and an anaesthetist. We visited South Auckland's Manukau Superclinic and Christchurch's Burwood Hospital, where elective units worked better than ours, then put a paper to management. Unfortunately, the manager, who was sympathetic, left for another post and the impetus died. Hospital doctors used to joke that the half-life of a good manager was about 18 months. They certainly turned over at an alarming rate and institutional memory left with them.

At Kenepuru I worked closely with a physician, Geoff Robinson. Sometime around 1999 Geoff proposed setting up a Māori health unit at the hospital: this arose from the high proportion of Māori patients we were treating. We decided to put our ideas to the popular and able minister of health, Annette King.

When we entered her office in the Beehive, the minister was surrounded by men in dark suits. We were not introduced. The minister was polite but detached. 'I've read your material, thank you. I need to hear your main concern. Please tell me.'

I briefly talked about Kenepuru being underused. 'I'm sure better use of the facilities there could help solve the congestion at Wellington Hospital and further your health aims,' I pronounced boldly. Geoff then talked about our proposal for a Māori health unit.

The interview was brief. 'I suggest you work with the senior Health Board administrators. I will alert them and arrange a meeting,' King said.

We trickled away. I felt deflated: I had already met with these administrators and got nowhere. At the subsequent meeting at Wellington Hospital, the scenario was familiar. You can imagine the result. My head hurt.

Scope for Surgery

The staff turnover at Kenepuru was low. Stable staff relationships made for good patient care. I greatly valued my theatre nurse colleagues. I worked alongside several chief theatre nurses and relationships were cordial. I remember only one occasion where things got tense. I was in theatre scrubs, it was getting late, and I was keen to get on to the next case. Yvonne, the theatre charge nurse and manager, was talking to the patient at length.

After waiting a while, I interrupted. 'Hello, Mrs Smith. Excuse me, Yvonne, can I please have a chat with Mrs Smith now? We need to get on with her operation.'

Yvonne ignored me and went on talking. I bristled. Why hadn't she talked to the patient earlier? I felt impatient and annoyed. A few minutes later I was able to talk with Mrs Smith but valuable operating time had ticked away.

While Mrs Smith was being wheeled into the anaesthetic room, I spoke to Yvonne in her office. 'Why didn't you allow me to get my turn with our patient after I had given you time to finish,' I blurted out. 'I felt ignored, and we were running out of time.'

Yvonne retorted, 'I was explaining the procedure to her. We nurses are the patients' advocates, you know.'

I was not going to let it go. 'Do you mean to say it's not my role to advocate too?'

'Well, we have a special responsibility,' Yvonne said.

I was aware surgeons no longer commanded automatic respect. I agreed with that: a sense of entitlement was the reason a few of my bosses had become arrogant. I expected to be questioned but this was going too far. I always saw myself as an advocate for my patients.

'Not acceptable to me, Yvonne,' I said. 'We're both advocates – I as much as you.' With that I stormed off into the theatre. We patched up our differences later.

Working in multiple hospital sites around greater Wellington, I was running myself ragged. Although I had a busy private practice, restricting my practice to private patients was out of the question. ACC funding for the large proportion of my patients meant I could treat them without cost but for others I was ambivalent about serving only those with the means to pay or privately insure themselves. I was, and still am, a major supporter of the public hospital system. There, I learnt my craft and could teach others. There, I could treat anybody regardless of their income and wealth. There, I could mix with a greater number and variety of medical colleagues and so keep up to date with new thinking.

A job based at Wellington Hospital, closer to home, would, I knew, require me to travel less and be less stressful. In 1990, an opportunity arose when Wellington's senior orthopaedic surgeon retired. Thinking I was well-qualified for the job, I applied.

Scope for Surgery

The senior appointments committee comprised leaders of the hospital's orthopaedic department, hospital management and other staff. On the evening after it had met to consider applications, Lindsay Haas, a neurologist and the chair of Combined Medical Staff, phoned me. 'Russell, your orthopaedic colleagues have screwed you,' he said.

I was taken aback. 'What do you mean?'

Then came the bombshell. 'Nothing in the advertisement stated that the board wanted someone with paediatric training, but they told us non-orthopods on the committee that's what is needed at Wellington Hospital.' The position had gone to a young surgeon who had just finished a fellowship in paediatric orthopaedic surgery in the United States.

I was stunned. 'How did the voting go?' I asked.

'There were two general surgeons there to consider another appointment, and bizarrely they were asked for their opinion. The whole thing was dodgy.'

This was huge. I valued the opinion of my peers and they had voted me down. I knew the young surgeon they had appointed. I liked him and thought him competent, but he had only just finished his training.

'What do you think I should do?' I said.

He didn't hesitate. 'Request a copy of the minutes – you have every right to see them. Then get yourself a professional industrial advocate and challenge the decision.'

The more I read of the meeting's minutes the more I saw how the appointment process had been skewed against me. My initial feeling of humiliation turned to disgust, but I was still ambivalent about challenging the decision. I imagined that if I were successful, I would have an uncomfortable time working alongside colleagues who had voted against me.

I sought advice from trusted friends, including my good friend from medical school days John Hutton, professor of obstetrics and gynaecology in Wellington. John said, 'You can't let this happen. You have to challenge the appointment.' Others said the same.

My challenge resulted in the establishment of a review appointments committee. I told the committee that I attended regular group meetings of orthopaedic surgeons practising in the wider Wellington area. At these there had been discussion for months about who might fill the vacant position, with no mention of the need for a surgeon with special expertise in dealing with orthopaedic conditions of childhood. Another surgeon on the Wellington team already had this expertise.

The job description stated that 'the appointee will be assisted to maintain special interests.' My advocate submitted to the committee: 'If what you want is a surgeon with a sub-specialty expertise not represented at Wellington Hospital, Mr Tregonning is the suitable candidate.'

I was the only surgeon in the wider Wellington region with a special interest in knee surgery.

The review committee decided in my favour. I was told it was the first time in the history of the Wellington Hospital that such a senior medical appointment had been changed. To my relief, when I took up the job my colleagues treated me perfectly well. I had no problem working harmoniously alongside them. Water under the bridge.

20.

Complications

OPERATIONS CAN HAVE UNDESIRABLE AND unintended complications. All surgeons have these. With the best will in the world, things can go wrong and patients suffer. We make mistakes and our systems fail. 'If a surgeon says he is having no complications, he is either lying or is not doing enough surgery' is an old adage. American surgeon Atul Gawande put it this way in his book *Complications: A Surgeon's Notes on an Imperfect Science*: 'We look for medicine to be an orderly field of knowledge and procedure. But it is not. It is an imperfect science, an enterprise of constantly changing knowledge, uncertain information, fallible individuals, and at the same time lives on the line.'

Complications

I remember few of my successful operations: the long training period and the learning curve with expert teachers made these unexceptional and routine. But when patients suffered major complications as a result of my surgery, it caused me much soul-searching. Vivid memories still haunt me decades later. I did a lot of surgery. The complications I describe here are only the more serious ones.

The first happened when I was a trainee in general surgery at Middlemore. The occasion was my old bête noir, stripping of the long saphenous vein. Varicose veins drain into this vein, which runs the length of the leg from ankle to groin. I had stopped feeling faint at the sight of the ghastly operation when I assisted my seniors, and was now learning to do it on my own.

The patient was an overweight middle-aged woman. She jabbed her finger to the back and side of her lower leg. 'I have an aching, burning pain in these ugly things. It's worse after I have been sitting or standing for long. I've tried raising my legs when I sit, castor oil, exercise, herbal creams, elastic bandages, the lot. They make my ankles swell. I want them out.'

Veins become varicosed when their valves are damaged, allowing blood to pool and vein walls to thin and swell. The patient's veins were dilated, ugly and tortuous. The skin on her ankle looked pigmented and fragile, as if it might ulcerate.

The process was to remove the channel into which these veins drained, the saphenous vein, by tying it off top and bottom, then ripping it out. Unfortunately, instead of tying the saphenous vein at its upper end, I tied off the large vein into which it drains, the femoral vein. This vein provides the main drainage from the whole leg. An obstruction causes major problems as blood pumped into the limb cannot properly escape.

I immediately recognised my mistake and called for help. I was lucky: my senior came quickly and made the repair. The patient suffered no harm but I did: I was devastated to have made such a basic error.

Nowadays, varicose veins can be treated with much less invasive procedures. Radiofrequency or laser ablation use heat or light to damage the inside of the vein, ultimately causing it to collapse and fade away. Another option for smaller varicose veins is sclerotherapy, which injects a solution that causes the vein to collapse.

My next general surgery run was at Auckland Hospital with the professor of surgery. He taught me that no surgeon is immune from mistakes. The professor was careful and meticulous, but during an operation to remove the parotid gland – the large salivary gland just in front of the ear – after expertly dissecting the vital facial nerve free to allow the gland to be easily removed, he inexplicably cut clean through it.

Complications

This is a well-known complication of this surgery. The facial nerve, running deep through the gland, is responsible for the movement of facial muscles. To make the disaster doubly tragic, the patient was the chief operating theatre nurse. Despite repair, she was left with a disfiguring paralysis of one side of her face. The professor was reminded of this every time he operated.

While working with this professor I was twice stung by a nasty feeling of incompetence. On one operation he had removed a cancerous portion of bowel, then sewed the two healthy ends of the bowel together, creating a joining line of stitches – an anastomosis. We now needed to make the suture line as watertight as possible. The professor punctured the stomach wall and inserted a balloon and tube into the stomach cavity.

'Okay, Russell, your turn now,' he said. 'Come over to this side of the table.' My job was to put a purse-string suture around the tube. The stitch could then be pulled tight to snug the wall around the tube and prevent stomach contents leaking into the abdominal cavity through the hole we'd created.

I put my curved needle down into the stomach wall, but too far. There was a muffled 'pop' as I pierced the balloon. The professor was understandably irritated. 'Too deep, too deep!' he said gruffly. 'I'll take over now.' I skulked back to the other side of the table.

Blood and Bone

My ego was bruised again soon afterwards. I had been given the main job of performing the bowel anastomosis after a bowel cancer removal. This time I pierced an artery.

The confidence of surgical trainees is fragile – mistakes can be catastrophic. Fortunately, neither of these was, but they helped drive me into orthopaedic surgery. Orthopaedic mistakes are distressing for all, particularly the patient, but they are seldom life-threatening.

Having an older brother who was an orthopaedic surgeon was useful. Garnet had always been a role model and once he saved my bacon. In 1978, when I was working at Tauranga Hospital as a senior registrar, I had little personal experience of spinal surgery. The senior surgeon with whom I was working did not do surgery for lumbar disc prolapses – the condition of the lower back commonly called a 'slipped disc'. The other senior surgeon also did no spinal surgery. Patients needing these operations were sent out of town.

I had assisted with and performed lumbar disc surgery a number of times during my training but never on my own. Nonetheless, I was confident I could operate on a gardener who came to us with a characteristic story. 'Six weeks ago I was in the garden,' he told me. 'I bent down to yank out a big clump of cocksfoot grass and felt a sudden jolt of pain like an electric shock go down my right leg.

Complications

It took my breath away. It was the worst pain I'd ever had.'

I asked him what happened after that. 'I saw my GP and rested up at home for a couple of weeks taking painkillers,' he said. 'I haven't returned to my job as the pain, tingling and weakness have not improved. It's excruciating when I cough or sneeze.'

When I asked if he'd experienced any disturbance to his bladder or bowel functions, a problem that can accompany this condition, he said no. If he had, it would have been more of a surgical emergency.

I examined him. There were signs of pressure on a nerve supplying his foot. An X-ray with injected dye confirmed that a piece of worn disc had moved backwards into the spinal canal and was pressing on the nerve. It all looked straightforward. I operated on his lower back. I saw no disc fragment: the spinal canal looked pristine. As I closed up I was mystified. What had I done wrong? I took another X-ray. This revealed my mistake: I had operated at the wrong level of the spine.

There is a high prevalence of wrong-level surgery in the lower back, even among experienced spinal surgeons. Both orthopaedic and neurosurgeons perform this type of surgery. A recent US study showed that half of all neurosurgeons will make a mistake with it during their career. One of the study's main recommendations was that the surgeon use an X-ray taken with the patient on the operating table, using a metal marker to identify the exact level before making the incision.

I had never seen this done but I knew that Garnet, experienced at spine surgery, had. He was working up the road at Middlemore. I rang him in distress. He told me to book the patient for re-operation on my next theatre list. 'Get the X-ray staff over for identification of the level before you go in,' he said. 'I'll come down to help.'

This was a major relief. My patient was relieved too; fortunately, he didn't blame me for the mistake. The re-operation went well and the patient made an excellent recovery. We kept the episode in the family. For every disc surgery I did after this I used the X-ray method.

Although surgeons know complications will happen, when we cause major trouble for a patient we often feel guilt and shame. British neurosurgeon Henry Marsh wrote in his book *Do No Harm*: 'When you approach a patient you have damaged it feels as if there is a force-field ... pushing you away from the patient's bed ... It is much easier to hurry past the patient without saying anything.'

Marsh's 'force-field' pushed strongly against me after I severely damaged a patient as a junior consultant at Kenepuru. Fred, a middle-aged man, was suffering from a condition affecting his low back that is caused by degenerative arthritis of the spine. Overgrowth of bone

Complications

(osteophytes or bone spurs), combined with a thickened ligament and the bulging of worn discs, takes up space. This constricts the spinal canal, a condition known as lumbar spinal stenosis. The result can be pain shooting down the legs, numbness and weakness. Walking some distance aggravates symptoms. So does arching the lower spine backwards. Resting and bending forward may relieve them.

Fred had the classic symptoms. 'I have really bad back pain,' he told me. 'Legs also. I only have to walk about 50 metres before developing an awful pain in my leg. Sometimes I also have tingling and weakness in my feet. I also sometimes get the pain in the morning, just standing and shaving under my chin as I look upwards.'

I asked him the routine questions about his pain. He said he could reduce it by sitting and bending forward. 'And I don't really understand it but walking uphill seems to be much less of a problem than walking downhill.' I explain that pain is relieved when we climb a hill because we bend our backs forwards.

The X-ray technique used dye injected into the spinal canal. It clearly showed that the space inside the spine was constricted. The aim of my operation was to nibble away the bone to make more space and relieve the pressure on the nerves.

I was sure to identify the levels with an X-ray in the operating theatre before I opened the skin. I then scraped the muscles off the bone attached to the back of the vertebrae with a sharp curved chisel we called the 'back scratcher' and used a bone-biting instrument – the 'back-biter' – to nibble away the bone. Because of the constriction this was difficult. The space was tight; the lower jaw of the instrument took up the little space available.

After the surgery I spoke to Fred, who had just woken up. 'Can you please lift your foot up at the ankle; lift your toes towards your nose.'

There was not a flicker of movement. I asked him to point his toes downwards. Again, no movement. 'Can you feel me scratch the top of your foot?' I asked. 'What about the sole?' Nothing.

My heart sank. I rang the neurosurgeon on call at Wellington Hospital. Within an hour we were back in theatre. We reopened the wound but there was no blood clot or bony spike constricting the nerves. I had damaged the blood supply to the nerve roots. There was nothing we could do to help.

I could barely make myself front up to Fred on our ward rounds. My profuse apologies seemed hollow. He didn't recover and was in a wheelchair when he visited me in the outpatients' department after discharge. He received financial compensation from ACC, but it was little for such a profound injury. I had wrecked this man's life. He was thereafter confined to a wheelchair. I have always felt extreme guilt; remembering the details and writing about it causes me grief over 30 years later.

There are 31 pairs of fragile and easily damaged motor and sensory nerve roots that come off the spinal cord. They connect the central nervous system – the brain and spinal cord – with the peripheral nervous system, the network of nerves that supplies the whole body, controlling sensation, movement and motor coordination. I never did enough spinal surgery to become entirely comfortable and therefore optimally proficient. I thought I would learn through performing the operations. This is a dilemma for all young surgeons: we have to start somewhere.

I didn't ever attempt the operation again, instead referring patients to more experienced colleagues. I did this for an increasing number of conditions where I felt I was not doing enough surgery to become, or remain, wholly competent.

In two other patients, during total hip replacement operations, I injured the longest and widest peripheral nerve, the sciatic. This nerve runs down the back of the thigh from inside the pelvis. Its branches extend down the leg. At its thickest, it is about two centimetres in diameter, the thickness of a little finger. It consists of two parts, of which the peroneal is at the greater risk of injury. This part of the nerve activates muscles in the leg responsible for pulling the foot upwards at the ankle, and outwards. It also allows sensation to be felt on some of the skin of the foot and lower leg. It was this I was responsible for injuring.

For the first of the surgeries, I was the operating surgeon. For the second I was the assistant, supervising my operating registrar. Although experienced, the registrar was still a trainee: I carried the can. In both cases the patients woke up from their hip replacements numb on the top and side of one foot and suffering the condition known as drop foot.

The healing of an injured nerve is unpredictable. Any return of function may be partial and take months. This makes waiting for recovery nerve-wracking for both patient and surgeon.

How had these injuries happened? Surgeons use several approaches to the hip to insert a prosthesis: from the front, the side and the back. Each has both strengths and possible complications. The posterior approach has a low complication rate but the highest rate of sciatic nerve injury; this is not surprising as the nerve runs over the back of the hip joint. Since I started work in Wellington I had used only the posterior approach, but I was always aware of the need to protect the sciatic nerve.

The technique of total hip replacement involves much stretching of soft tissues to allow access. This is particularly difficult when the patient is obese. The operative field becomes deeper and deeper as the surgeon cuts through a thick layer of subcutaneous fat. Keeping the thick tissue edges apart and operating at the bottom of a deep wound is hazardous for the patient and stressful for the surgeon.

While operating on an obese patient one day, I got frustrated. 'Where the hell is the bone? I know it must be down here somewhere,' I exclaimed. We wrestled with the limb to dislocate the joint – more stretching and bad language. I guiltily checked with the anaesthetist to make sure the patient was asleep and couldn't hear my offensive remarks. I have read that swearing helps relieve stress. I discovered that in theatre long ago. It doesn't have to be strongly worded, but it does have to be vehement.

The instruments required to perform hip replacements would fit well into a medieval torture chamber and the theatre resembles an abattoir. Retractors that keep the soft tissues apart have metal spikes to be hammered into bone, wide metal blades, ratcheted self-retaining rakes, and hooks. We prod the wound with a blunt-nosed sucker to clear blood and irrigation fluid so we can see. We burn soft tissue using high-frequency electric currents – a process known as diathermy – to cut through tissue and coagulate blood vessels to reduce bleeding. There is a strong smell of burning flesh.

We wield serious power tools to saw and drill bone. Sometimes I get blood, fat or bone dust in my eye around my specs. It stings. A strong stream of saline solution rids the wound of blood and bone fragments, flushing the joint and cleansing it. We suck and mop the raw bony surfaces dry. Finally, we anchor the new joint pieces. If cementing, we force liquid methyl methacrylate cement into bone with a syringe. The cement reaches high temperatures that may damage the bone, so we dribble cold saline solution over it as it hardens. Then, whether cementing or not, we quickly and vigorously hammer the artificial joint into place.

Sciatic nerve injury can come about in many ways during this controlled mayhem, but this devastating complication is relatively rare, reportedly happening in only about 1.5 percent of primary hip replacement operations, although the real incidence may be higher as surgeons tend to under-report complications. It occurs more often in revision surgery as scarring from the original wound sticks tissues together and distorts the anatomy.

During the two injury cases, my assistant and I had taken all the usual precautions to protect the nerve. We were unaware of the injuries while we were operating and didn't ever discover the causes. Understandably, both patients were disappointed and, I'm sure, lost faith in my competence.

Neither injury got better with time. I fitted each patient with a special device to hold up their foot and prevent the slapping and high-stepping gait a sufferer must use to clear their dropped foot from the ground while walking. With one patient I operated to transfer a tendon from behind her ankle to the top of her foot; this gave her some power to lift her foot without the device.

From then on, hip replacement surgery made me anxious. I couldn't relax after surgery until I was sure my patient's nerve was working well. I would sometimes go into the recovery room more than once while the person slowly recovered consciousness, itching to test their sciatic nerve function and assure myself all was well. I was greatly relieved when a fully conscious patient pulled up their foot at my request. I could then share his or her relief and bask in the pleasure of a job well done.

Sadly, I suffered a nerve injury when my own hip was replaced. I knew the surgeon was skilful; I had observed his work close up. Despite this the operation, using the side approach, turned out to be complicated. My hip still causes me pain and 'snapping'. Wanting to rule out a detached tendon, I travelled to Melbourne to consult a surgeon who had operated on hundreds of hip joints using the keyhole method. He confirmed the diagnosis of nerve injury.

Mistakes are distressing, some more than others. I still suffer angst about Daniel, a 14-year-old boy who presented with a painful wrist.

'My wrist started to hurt a couple of weeks ago,' he

told me. 'I thought I must have knocked it when I was out biking. I don't remember any fall or other real injury.'

I asked if the pain was worse when he used his hand. 'No,' he said, 'it seems to hurt all the time, even when I'm doing nothing – in bed at night, particularly.'

Pain at rest in a young limb without arthritis and with no history of injury rang alarm bells. When I examined Daniel's wrist, it looked normal and was only a little tender to the touch. The joint moved normally. But the X-ray showed an area of destroyed bone in his lower radius, the thicker of the two forearm bones. Its appearance told me it was rapidly growing. It looked like a malignant tumour, probably an osteosarcoma. This condition can be lethal when it spreads through the body.

I quickly operated and took out a small piece of the tumour. The pathologist reported a serious malignancy. I discussed the findings with him. He was certain of the diagnosis.

The limb looked normal, with none of the usual signs of advanced disease. There was no grotesque deformity, no swelling, no signs of trauma, no discolouration or ulceration of skin. And Daniel could use the arm well.

At a clinical meeting that week I showed my senior orthopaedic colleagues the X-rays and biopsy result. The patient's age, clinical presentation and radiology all suggested a dangerous tumour. The decision was unanimous.

Complications

I must quickly amputate his arm. The only question was whether I should do so below or above the elbow. Most favoured above the elbow.

I hated telling Daniel and his parents what I had to do and why. Daniel was stoic. About three weeks after the operation, when his wound had healed well and he had visited the artificial-limb fitters, I opened my mail to a bombshell. Unbeknown to me, the Wellington pathologist had sent the biopsy specimen to a leading American hospital that specialised in bone tumours. Its pathologists had diagnosed an unusual but probably benign tumour.

I was stunned. The pathologist had expressed no real doubt about his diagnosis of malignancy or told me he was requesting an overseas opinion. I dreaded having to tell Daniel.

Some years later he came to me for an unrelated injury. He seemed to be coping well, but he didn't like his artificial arm and didn't use it. He didn't seem to blame me, at least not to my face. He appeared to have accepted his fate. I never have.

21.

Dangerous Bacteria

INFECTION IS AN EVER-PRESENT THREAT in surgery. Normal skin is teeming with organisms. As soon as it is breached with an incision, these organisms and those on clothing and elsewhere in the environment can contaminate the wound.

Before doctors understood that bacteria caused infection and how important it was to sterilise everything, surgery was hazardous. Even today, our routine of painting skin with powerful antiseptics and isolating the operative field using sterile drapes doesn't rid the patient's skin of all organisms. Operating teams thoroughly disinfect their hands, don sterile gloves and wear gowns, but infection remains a constant worry.

Dangerous Bacteria

Much activity in hospitals is aimed at lessening the incidence of surgical site infections, SSIs. For a short time after I first entered an orthopaedic theatre in the late '60s, I saw surgeons using the 'no touch' technique. Only sterile instruments entered the wound. Now we have improved theatre sterility, movements of people in and out of theatre are minimised, and operating teams often double-glove.

Sepsis, infection, is still the most common surgical complication. The two most feared types in orthopaedics are infection of the joint (septic arthritis) and infection in the bone (osteomyelitis). Both can cause pain, fever and shivering. Inflammation may make the part warm to the touch. To halt the risk of permanent damage, urgent treatment with antibiotics is required. The infected joint requires drainage and irrigation. The joint, and sometimes the bone also may require surgical cleaning out. In extreme cases the sepsis can lead to amputation and even death.

Over my practising lifetime, antibiotics have been increasingly used to try to prevent infection. When implanting large foreign material such as artificial joints and fixation devices into a patient, we routinely inject heavy doses of antibiotics into their bloodstream. These enter the body's tissues before the skin is cut: we want to make the internal body environment as hostile as possible for bacteria. Nowadays, a major problem is the emergence of antibiotic-resistant bacteria.

Blood and Bone

The youngest patient on whom I performed a knee replacement was Brendon, aged 20. Brendon worked as a garage attendant. His knee had been destroyed when he was 19 because of a staphylococcus septic arthritis. A few months before he came to me, he had sought advice from a surgeon because his knee was sore. The surgeon had performed an arthroscopy. Brendon's new problem was an unusually painful scar at the site where the arthroscope had been inserted.

My registrar cut out the scarred area, going down into the joint to completely remove it. It was a minor operation and Brendon was discharged from hospital the same day.

A week later he again presented at my clinic. 'A couple of days ago my knee swelled up and became very painful,' he said. 'I can't sleep because of the pain and I've been feeling unwell. Mostly I feel really hot, although sometimes I feel cold and shiver like mad.'

I examined him. He was clearly very sick: his temperature was high and his knee was swollen and hot. Attempting to move it caused him considerable pain.

I diagnosed septic arthritis. We sucked fluid off his knee using a needle but didn't wait for the laboratory result: his clinical condition and the nasty-looking fluid was enough. We started intravenous antibiotics, which we knew would kill most staphylococci. We took him to the operating theatre, opened the knee and thoroughly washed out the infection.

Dangerous Bacteria

Although Brendon's knee settled down in hospital, after he was discharged our systems failed him. We should have followed up after a few days. Instead, he didn't come back to us for two weeks. He had been suffering little pain – the inflammation was no doubt dampened by the antibiotics he was still taking – but when we removed the knee splint it was clear the infection had not been eliminated. His X-ray was alarming. There was an almost complete loss of clear space between the bones: the infection had destroyed most of the cartilage.

We took him to theatre and washed his knee out again, but over the following months he developed severe bone-on-bone pain. Despite the risk of a prosthesis becoming infected, we felt there was no choice but to insert a total knee replacement. We used industrial doses of antibiotics, both intravenously and in the cement holding the knee replacement in place. The result was not perfect. Brendon still experienced some pain, but it was tolerable.

International data shows that nine out of ten total knee replacements last for 20 years. Young patients have a much greater risk of failure than older people because they tend to be more active and so put more stress on their replaced joints. The latest New Zealand data shows replacements in people under 40 failed about three times earlier than in people aged about 70. (The average age for patients receiving total knee replacements is 68.)

Brendan will almost certainly need his knee replaced, maybe multiple times. There's also a risk of his latest or a subsequent knee replacement becoming infected: bacteria in bone can remain dormant for years then suddenly wake up and cause trouble.

Staphylococcus bacteria (the name is commonly shortened to Staph or S.) live on human skin and usually cause no problem. Brendan's knee was infected with S. aureus (aureus is Latin for gold, the colour of the Staph colonies when grown in the lab). This is found in 20 to 30 percent of people, in noses and other moist places such as armpits and groins. It can cause skin infections such as boils and impetigo and is the most common cause of serious bone and joint infection.

The less virulent S. epidermidis is found on everybody's skin, wet or dry. It causes infection when it gets inside the body and settles around an implant such as an artificial joint. Bacteria stick to the surface of the implant and produce a layer of polysaccharide, proteins and adhesives. This 'biofilm' allows the bacteria to hunker down, protected from extinction by antibiotics and the body's immune defences.

This complication marred an early success story for my patient Allan, a 67-year-old man with a painful osteoarthritic knee. Allan was fit, with no conditions that might predispose him to infection. His total knee replacement was routine and went well. After surgery and rehabilitation, he had no pain. 'Last week I did two rounds of golf,' he told me. 'It's great to be active again. I don't notice the knee.'

Many months later he hobbled into the clinic with a stick. His knee was painful and swollen. I had that sinking feeling. 'I'm very sorry to see you like this, Allan,' I said. 'What happened?'

He couldn't remember having an injury or sudden mishap. 'It just came out of the blue,' he said. 'The pain got worse and worse and now the knee's starting to give way on me. I think the thing may have worked loose. Perhaps I twisted too much during my golf swing.'

But it wasn't golf that was the cause of Allan's pain: the fluid I aspirated from his knee grew staphylococcus epidermidis in the lab. An X-ray showed the bone around his metal implant was being destroyed.

In New Zealand fewer than one percent of knee replacements need re-operation for any reason in the first 12 months after surgery. When they do need fixing, it is usually because of deep infection. If this occurs within the first few weeks after surgery, it can be possible to keep the knee replacement by removing the infected joint lining, bone and other tissue, washing the whole area, replacing the plastic part of the joint (it is separate from the metal part and removable) and putting the patient on a long-term course of antibiotics. But if the infection strikes months or years later, as it did for Allan, there's no option but to replace the artificial joint.

This is a long arduous process. Allan had multiple surgeries, prolonged time in hospital, and massive quantities of antibiotics – first intravenously and for months afterwards by pills.

In the first operation I removed the artificial joint, together with the damaged and dead bone and cement and washed the soft tissues with saline. There was now a gaping hole between the bones. I filled this with a thick disc of bone cement that would keep the soft tissues out to their correct length. It was laden with antibiotic, which would slowly leach into the surrounding bone and soft tissue. However, the filler prevented knee movement. Methods developed since then use spacers, which allow some motion.

After two months we took fluid from Allan's knee and sent it to the lab. When we were satisfied the knee was sterile, we operated again – this time to insert a new joint. This had to be much larger to fill the hole created by the removal of the original and the infected bone around it. The next problem was how to properly fix it into healthy bone. We attached thick metal stems to the prosthesis and bored out the shafts of the femur and tibia to allow us to secure these stems, a major procedure. Allan regained only about half of his knee movement and had continuing discomfort. He didn't get back to his golf. Nobody was happy.

Surgeons in New Zealand warn patients of all possible major complications so that if one occurs it should come as no surprise. But of course it always does. Unlike in the United States, most patients don't sue hospitals or medical professionals. Some do complain to their hospital, district health board or other body such as the Accident Compensation Corporation or the Health and Disability Commissioner. The commissioner may refer serious misdemeanours to the New Zealand Medical Council. Conditions can be placed on a doctor's practice. The doctor's name can be made public. In the worst cases the doctor can be removed from the medical register and so barred from practising medicine.

Although I caused my share of complications, I was only once entangled with the Health and Disability Commissioner. Three months before seeing me, Brenda, a 25-year-old netballer, had ruptured her Achilles, the strong tendon at the back of the ankle that joins the calf muscle to the heel. She described how her injury happened. 'I suddenly pushed off to chase the ball from a standing start. I heard a "crack". It felt as if somebody had hit me at the back of my ankle, but I looked back and there was nobody there. I was in great pain and had to limp off the court.'

There are two treatment options for this disabling injury. If the patient gets to a doctor within the first 48 hours, before the calf muscle has retracted permanently upwards, a plaster cast may work. The patient's ankle will be immobilised, with the foot pushed down at the toes and up at the heel – the 'equinus' position. (Equinus means 'as in a horse': horses walk on tiptoe.) This allows the two ends of tendon to approach close to each other and the tendon to heal as near to the original length as possible. This was the treatment Brenda had received from a surgeon.

The alternative would have been surgery to join the two ends of the tendon. This is necessary if treatment is late. Delay is likely to lead to shortening of the calf muscle and lengthening of the healed tendon.

Each treatment has pros and cons. Surgery means a stronger tendon of more normal length but a higher chance of complications, such as infections and the wound breaking down. The soft tissue covering the Achilles tendon is thin, with little subcutaneous fat. Surgery can disturb the tenuous blood supply to the skin.

Putting the ankle in a cast means a greater chance of a weaker, longer Achilles tendon, which may rupture again. This is what had happened to Brenda.

I could feel a large gap between the two ends of the tendon. I operated, using a well-known reconstruction method. This involved turning down a strip of tendon from above, bridging the gap, and attaching it to the tendon stump below. I didn't much like the bulk of the reconstructed tendon: the skin was a little tight when I closed it, but I judged it to be acceptable.

Brenda was pleased. After her discharge from hospital she wrote me a letter expressing gratitude for the treatment, which she rated as excellent. However, her pleasure was short-lived. Some days after the operation she reported to Christchurch Hospital. She was in pain. The wound had broken down due to an infection. The hospital operated to clean out the infected material; this included removal of the tendon strip, which was now dead.

I went from saint to sinner. She complained about me and her complaint reached the Health and Disability Commissioner. The essence was that I had failed to treat her with prophylactic antibiotics. The commissioner sought an opinion from an orthopaedic surgeon in another city. The surgeon stated that for a clean soft-tissue operation without insertion of substantial foreign material, prophylactic antibiotics were not obligatory. I thought the cause may have been an overtight closure, but infection can occur in any surgical wound despite all precautions taken. It may have just been bad luck.

I was told by Wellington Hospital management that I must attend a meeting in a few days, where I was to apologise to Brenda. I had no choice of time and day. I had no problem with expressing my extreme regret for what had happened, but the meeting was scheduled to be on my operating theatre day. I would have had to cancel surgery for several patients who had waited months for their operations. I was in a bind. I decided to treat my patients as scheduled. I apologised for not being able to attend the meeting and explained why.

This occurred shortly after the Health and Disability Commission had been set up. I was cited by the first commissioner as having transgressed the Health and Disability code as I had failed to attend the meeting. A colleague on the Medical Council later told me confidentially that some of the early decisions by the commission were considered dubious. He assured me there would be no repercussions. He was right. The Medical Council was untroubled when I next applied to renew my practising certificate. I had learnt a lesson both about bureaucracy and, more valuably for future patients, my surgical technique.

The story had a happy ending. About twelve months later I saw Brenda in my outpatients' clinic. To my surprise and her satisfaction, her tendon had regenerated to almost normal form and function.

Shortly after this, a colleague of mine had a less fortunate experience: he operated on the wrong knee. Realising his mistake while still in theatre, he then operated on the correct knee. The patient complained. The commission found the doctor in breach of the code of conduct and referred the case to the Medical Practitioners Disciplinary Tribunal. The tribunal dismissed a charge of professional misconduct but released the surgeon's name to the media. The incident was deemed a 'system error' but the tribunal stressed that the doctor was primarily responsible. The patient was awarded financial compensation and the costs of her treatment.

New Zealand's unique no-fault accident compensation scheme provides money and support to citizens, residents and temporary visitors who suffer personal injuries. One of its categories is 'treatment injury'. If a claim is accepted, the ACC may pay or contribute to the costs of treatment, rehabilitation and compensation for misdiagnosis, surgical errors and other treatment-related injuries.

In many countries, most notably the United States, doctors may be sued. The cost of insurance for doctors is huge and drives up their fees. Injured patients may have a long wait for legal action and resolution. If eventually successful, they may be awarded huge sums. However, it is like a lottery and few get compensated. Most get nothing.

In New Zealand patients get compensated quickly, albeit with smaller pay-outs. The scheme started in 1974, my first year of orthopaedic training. Before that, as a house surgeon, I had seen senior doctors often called away to court to give evidence in workers' compensation cases. I had heard their frustration with what they saw as a waste of their time. Often, they would have a long wait at the court before being called to give evidence. Our operating lists at the hospital were sometimes disrupted because of their absences. The ACC system brought advantages for patients and doctors alike.

My colleagues' experience and my own brush with the Health and Disability Commission prompted me to improve the information I gave my patients before elective surgery. I wanted them to know and accept that, no matter how fervently I wished for success and how carefully I acted, my operating on them would expose them to risk. I prepared a short information sheet to be included in the patient record. It described the complications possible with orthopaedic procedures. There are many, so I listed in simple language only the most common, adding that there also were other, rarer complications.

One patient expressed alarm at the opening paragraph of the sheet – in essence a modification of the concept, well-known to surgeons, that 'there is no surgical operation known to man that can't make you worse'. He considered it too brutal and offered to rewrite it. I rapidly accepted. He couched the gist of my message in gentler, more expert language.

The alarmed patient was Roger Robinson, professor

of English at Victoria University and a champion runner. I had first met him when we both spoke at a running event in Nelson in the 1980s; he was the entertaining after-dinner speaker, while I had been invited to talk about the mundane topic of knee injuries in runners. Our acquaintance had been short – on the ten-kilometre run, he had quickly become a dot in the distance.

When I saw him again in 2011, Roger had had a painful osteoarthritic knee for 15 years. Recently, it had stopped him running. I replaced it with an Oxford uni. Later his other knee also wore out. He was then living in the United States and got a total knee replacement from an American surgeon. He named his knee replacements after his surgeons: 'Russell' for his right knee and 'Mark' for his left.

Roger was not a quitter. In an article in *PodiumRunner* magazine in May 2020 he was quoted saying, 'One time I believed that it was all over, when knee replacement surgery officially meant I would never run again. Wrong. In ten years since then, I've run 91 races from one mile to half-marathon.'

The 'official' word had come from me. It was the standard advice orthopaedic surgeons gave patients with new knees: avoid jarring the knee by running. Our logic was that the bond between the bone and the artificial joint would probably fail over time and the joint would loosen.

We advised our patients to keep active with low-impact sports such as cycling, swimming and gym.

In 2017 Roger wrote an article in *Runner's World* entitled 'Here's How I Returned to Racing After Knee Replacement: A lifelong runner finds new satisfaction in running – and opens his surgeon's eyes to the possibilities.' Of his return to running he said he 'sort of forgot, and tried a little running, just ten paces to begin with ...'

He described his slow build-up to a return to competitive running. 'In the second year I tried a few races, still walking any downhills or uneven footing, and came in dead last, one time behind some women chatting as they walked with strollers, another time after losing a memorable duel with a nine-year-old girl.'

The article interested the American orthopaedic community. In 2018, the Academy of Orthopaedic Surgeons gave Roger an award. 'It's important for us ... to recognise journalists for the work they do to inform the public about life-changing musculoskeletal treatments used to improve patients' lives,' the president said.

Since my advice to Roger, one study has shown that running with knee and hip replacements does no harm and may be of some benefit. In 2016, the Oxford group compared post-operative results for high-activity patients with those for low-activity patients. The study included all types of sport. The high-activity patients were more satisfied with the results of their operation, although the difference was not statistically significant. The researchers concluded: 'This suggests there is no justification to advise patients to restrict their activities.' However, the follow-up period was only about six years, and the authors added a cautious rider. 'As revision due to polyethylene wear [degradation of the implant] and osteolysis [bone destruction] may occur in the second and third decades of use, further follow-up of these patients is required to assess long-term consequences of increased activity level.'

So while Roger opened my eyes to the possibilities, the jury is still out on the long-term effects of running. A surgeon's responsibility is to report the best evidence available, describe known complications, and let the patient decide.

22.

Passing On the Baton

AN IMPORTANT AND ENJOYABLE PART of my job has been sharing knowledge with patients about their conditions. Patients often wait a long time for an appointment; there is pressure to get as many through the consulting room as quickly as possible. I resisted this and always gave new patients a full half hour. I liked sharing their X-rays and answering questions brought on by their previous consultation with family, friends and other 'experts', including, latterly, Dr Google.

There are many traps for patients, particularly those suffering the pain of arthritis. On print and digital media well-known figures, frequently sportspeople or media celebrities, extol the virtues of non-prescription drugs, dietary supplements and other potions claiming to miraculously cure or alleviate pain. The words 'natural health and nutrition' regularly appear. These paid promoters are driven by money and almost all have no medical knowledge.

Even pharmacists may have large stacks of 'joint food' or fish oil enticingly displayed in their shops. The producers of these 'remedies' take advantage of the fact that with common wear-and-tear arthritis there are periods of strong pain but also relatively pain-free times. If a drug, supplement or ointment is used just before a natural remission period, it will tend to get the credit. Reputable trials have shown that the only 'joint food' with any effect is glucosamine. Some people taking it report relief from pain and stiffness, particularly for knee arthritis; others report no benefit. No supplements give permanent relief or prevent or cure osteoarthritis.

I have always been interested in the academic side of surgery: assessing the results of operations, passing on lessons learnt, reporting to colleagues. Doctors are competitive: we test each other on our knowledge. One-upmanship is endemic. At conferences we vigorously debate the pros and cons of diagnostic methods, treatment methods and the desirability of operating, and if so how.

Thinking on disorders of the human skeleton and its

attached soft tissues and methods of treatment changes rapidly; worldwide, researchers publish thousands of orthopaedic papers every year. Doctors are required to keep up-to-date. Coping with this constant mutating body of knowledge is a struggle but stimulating. Orthopaedic journals have always been at my bedside. I read at night, no doubt hastening my drifting off to sleep. I count bones, not sheep. I haven't ever got to 206, the number of bones in the adult human.

I have also enjoyed testing junior colleagues' ability to diagnose and treat patients, probing their knowledge and encouraging them to think logically. There is a well-practised ritual. Junior doctors present clinical cases, outlining the patients' stories and the results of their physical examination and investigations. Senior doctors then assess their ability to interpret the history, the examination findings and the lab, X-ray and scan results. The information is shared with others at the session, with X-rays and scans flashed up on a screen. The junior doctors are asked what further investigations they might order, and what action they might take to fix or alleviate the problem. Everyone is invited to participate in a free-for-all exchange of opinion and information, sometimes combative but usually good-natured.

On one occasion I was running a teaching session about bone tumours. These tumours are not common compared with injuries and arthritis, but it's vital to diagnose them early. I outlined the history of a patient I had treated. 'She was a female, aged 16, who complained of pain in the front of her right knee and lower thigh. She had had it for three months. Nothing seemed to help. The pain was a constant dull ache, getting gradually worse and now disturbing her sleep. The blood tests her GP had ordered were all normal.' I asked those in the room, 'What else do you want to ask me?'

One registrar asked about the patient's general health. Was there are past or family history of illness?

'There was no history of injury, and the family history was negative,' I said.

What had I found when I examined the patient, another asked.

'Her general health was excellent. She walked normally – no limp. The knee and lower thigh exams were unremarkable.'

A registrar asked, 'What about your examination of hip and spine?' This doctor knew that a spinal, or more commonly a hip, problem might radiate pain to the knee. This is so-called 'referred pain'.

'Good question.' I said. 'As you suggest, we must always think of something north of the knee in a case like this where the knee looks normal. I was recently referred a patient whose surgeon had removed the kneecap when the cause of the patient's pain was a hip arthritis, which the surgeon had missed. That patient had had no groin pain. All his pain was in the front of the knee.'

I asked another registrar, 'What X-rays will you order?'

'X-rays of the knee, pelvis and hip,' she replied.

I flashed the X-rays up on the screen. 'Please come up, inspect them and comment.'

She thought the X-rays were normal and we agreed.

'So what now?' I asked a house surgeon. A blank look. 'Anybody?'

A registrar's hand shot up. 'What about a radioactive technetium bone scan?'

'And for the rest here, what is that?'

'A bone scan images the metabolic activity of the skeleton,' he replied. 'The technetium is injected into a vein. It is taken up in the skeleton where the bone metabolism is high, such as in a tumour where the cells are dividing rapidly.'

I showed them the scan. In the middle of the thigh bone, a small area was lit up like a light bulb. I put up an X-ray of the whole femur. At the same position in the femur as in the scan there was an area of dense white bone about the size of a small fingernail. The X-rays of the knee and hip had missed the vital area.

'What are the possible causes here?' I asked a senior trainee. I knew he was a walking textbook: he was about to sit his final surgeon's ticket exam and had been studying hard.

Passing on the Baton

'It's an osteoid osteoma,' he said confidently. 'You can see a small area of low-density black bone in the middle of the dense white area. It's diagnostic of a rather rare benign tumour that needs removing.'

He was right. I told the meeting I had operated and removed the tumour. The lab report had confirmed the diagnosis. As with almost all patients with this condition, the pain had disappeared.

I valued the rapport with the young registrars who worked with me for six months at a time. The relationship of consultant and trainee is close in medicine. Good communication is essential. The consultant must provide an atmosphere that encourages trainees to ask for help: firm guidance rather than rigid requirements; praise for good work; gentle instruction when there are problems; and practical help, such as going to the hospital at night to help with road accident multiple trauma cases.

Sometimes in theatre when there was a new problem to solve, I would bounce ideas off senior trainees. 'What approach is Mr Y using these days – going in from the back or front or side?' 'How would Mr X deal with this situation?' Or perhaps, 'What do you reckon will be the better fixation here: rod or plate?'

It is vital that doctors educate themselves throughout their careers. The Medical Council and other bodies require practising doctors to undertake continuing professional development. For surgeons like me, this included auditing my operations and complication rates.

As I became more experienced at presenting my work I enlisted trainees to help with research. We assessed results of my operations and compared them with those recorded in the literature, or analysed data about knee replacements recorded in New Zealand's National Joint Registry. One of us would then present to our colleagues.

With my own talks I was excited, but at the same time nervous about failing in front of my colleagues. Time spent assessing patients, collating the results, then creating the talk meant hours of work per slide. For most presentations, the time allowed was seven minutes. The temptation for a rookie was to try and fit in too much information. I fell into this trap. At my first presentation to a national audience, the chair whispered urgently in my ear, 'Time's up. Stop now!'

The terror of more reprimands made me learn fast. I rehearsed and precisely timed all subsequent presentations. I progressed to short sharp messages on uncrowded slides with plenty of pictures.

Once, in the early '80s, I felt I'd failed as a teacher. I was operating on a patient with an unstable torn meniscal fragment. The operation was being videoed live to demonstrate arthroscopy techniques. My colleagues watched and listened from another room while I talked through my technique. After I detached a portion of the meniscus, I lost control of the fragment and couldn't find it again – the mouse-like piece had sneaked into a hole. I couldn't see my colleagues' reaction, but their questions and comments gradually died down and then there was silence. They had gone off for tea.

In 2000 I volunteered for orthopaedic work in Vietnam as part of a New Zealand government aid programme. I helped teach orthopaedic surgeons, spending an eye-opening three weeks at Binh Dinh General Hospital in Quy Nhon, a city of about 200,000 people on the south-central coast. A New Zealand surgical team had worked at the hospital since 1963, the first, and eventually the last New Zealand commitment made during what the Americans call the Vietnam War and the Vietnamese the American War. Our soldiers left in December 1973; the surgical team carried on till 1975 just before the North Vietnamese tanks rolled into Saigon. As well as treating civilian, war and accident casualties, the team had trained Vietnamese medics and nurses in all aspects of modern hospital medicine, including maternity, paediatrics and public health promotion.

New Zealanders like us, visiting 25 years later, were treated with affection: unlike the Americans, our wartime team had treated injured Viet Cong soldiers. After the country opened to the outside world in 1995, surgeon

Allan Panting (the leader) and our group of four doctors and two nurses had been among the first New Zealand medical teams invited back by the Vietnamese to volunteer their services.

The conditions in the orthopaedic ward were hard to believe. There were often two patients to a bed. There were no curtains for privacy. Flimsy splints were used instead of traction for fractured limbs, sometimes for a long time. There was little early surgery; fractures were uniting while patients' limbs were short and bent. Relatives washed and provided meals for their injured family members and their stuff was strewn about the wards. There were no handbasins, so nurses changed dressings without adequate hygiene.

There was no properly funded public health system. Much of the delay in surgery was because relatives had to rally around to fund it. Many surgeons had jobs outside the hospital to bolster their meagre pay.

I was in for more surprises in the operating theatre. The room was hot and lacked air conditioning. The ancient broken operating table was set so low I had to bend uncomfortably. Because of the long delays, many long-bone fractures were in an advanced stage of healing; we had to unpick the healing tissue to align them properly and pull them out to their normal length. It was hard, sweaty work. I prayed my perspiration dripping into limb wounds would not cause infection.

Passing on the Baton

It was our policy to help and guide the local surgeons, rather than perform the operations ourselves. With complex cases the surgeons sometimes resisted and wanted us to take the lead. On these occasions I felt I had to agree: the language barrier made merely guiding a near impossibility. But in another way the operations were simple. The patients were thin, making for easy access to the bones.

Amid the chaos, the able Vietnamese surgeons worked with primitive technology. Most of the metal they used was pre-loved – or, more accurately, pre-lived: it had previously resided in patients in other countries. If deeply implanted metalware doesn't irritate a patient's tissues we tend to leave it in place, but if it does we remove plates, screws and rods. Those that are undamaged by the removal process and mechanically still sound can be satisfactorily reused, although we never recycle them in New Zealand.

Pre-warned, I took some of this hardware with me from my own operations. Before surgery we would open a drawer and choose from the jumble of assorted bits and pieces, holding up a used metal rod or plate against the X-ray of a broken bone to estimate the length and width needed. Often the part was only approximately suitable. It would then be sterilised. If it wasn't quite right, too bad and too late – we had made our choice.

Then came the screws. There were no trays with a vast number of sizes to choose from, as at home. New

Zealanders have a reputation for being good number-eight-wire technologists. If there was no screw of the length required, we employed a long-handled bolt cutter to create one from a longer screw.

It was impossible to get X-rays in theatre. A mobile unit had been brought from the old New Zealand military hospital at Whenuapai, but before our visit staff in the radiology department had unplugged it, moved it and hard-wired it into their department. They felt their need was greater than ours.

We treated many road trauma victims. It was not hard to see why. On the roads around the town there was a crush of bicycles and small motorbikes. Sometimes the motorbikes carried huge loads: a whole family, including children; a live pig or two in crates; building material or furniture. There were no helmets and head injuries were common. There seemed to be few rules and cars passed each other at high speed. When travelling I often saw vehicles approaching on the wrong side of the road, barely missing us by swerving at the last minute.

The Vietnamese people were still emerging from the devastation of the war, which had ended just a generation before. I felt embarrassed that New Zealand had played a part in the conflict. The Americans had killed about two million civilians and left the country a bombed-out defoliated wreck. Their government had then led trade embargoes, denied reconstruction aid, and plunged the population into poverty. With my rusty fifth-form French, I tried to apologise to the older people who spoke French for our country having supported the Americans. They were cordial and generous. They seemed not to blame New Zealand, at least to my face. At the end of my stay I went on a short guided tour. I found a beautiful country and gentle resilient people. I felt I had gained more than I had given.

On my return home I toyed with volunteering again, but reluctantly decided the discomfort of operating in such primitive conditions was too much for me. I wished I had volunteered when I was younger, with a stronger back and more energy. The Vietnam experience remains a vivid memory. I am grateful to have worked there and gained first-hand knowledge of how unequal our world is, how cruel humans are to each other, and how privileged New Zealanders are.

I had begun to feel burnout in Vietnam. When I returned, I found being on call after hours increasingly onerous but felt a responsibility to be present when there were difficult acute trauma cases for operation. I reasoned that my name was on the end of the bed, so the buck stopped with me. I would get out of bed, wipe the sleep from my eyes, drive through the night, mask and scrub up, and don gown and gloves.

A major driver for this night work was the lack of operating time during the day. We performed surgery on acutely injured patients after hours to avoid having to cancel cases the next day. This has changed. Most major hospitals now have daytime 'acute' operating lists, patients having been temporarily stabilised the night before. In this way, fresh surgical teams work on the trauma patients, rather than tired on-call surgeons and night nursing teams who may be unfamiliar with the huge inventory of orthopaedic surgical devices.

There were other reasons for my angst. Pamela and I had joined the executive of a community organisation called Waterfront Watch and met many interesting, active and inspiring people. Our aim was to stop the Wellington City Council allowing the construction of about 20 high-rise buildings on the waterfront between the city and the harbour – a potential abomination we called The Great Wall of Wellington. I was appointed to an official citizens' advisory group. It was frustrating fighting our own city council. Although Waterfront Watch and its sister organisation Chaffers Park – Make It Happen! succeeded in mobilising public opinion and the wall of buildings was at least partially stopped, the campaign added to my level of stress.

I began the familiar pattern of waking early and feeling tense and low, particularly in the mornings. By evening

Passing on the Baton

I usually felt fine again. By now I knew these were the classical symptoms of anxiety and depression. I sought treatment. My psychiatrist, Pete Ellis, was a lifesaver. After some weeks of taking anti-depressants I was feeling better. I spent time easing back into the operating theatre, assisting a colleague. Ellis started to push me. 'Don't you think it's time to start operating on your own now, Russell?' I had stage fright. 'I can't trust myself,' I said. He egged me on. 'Well, I'd trust you to operate on me'. That did it. With each operation I gained in confidence.

My rising discomfort with night work and tiredness on days after I'd operated at night seemed, however, to be telling me it was time for a change of job. I wondered about a management role, but quickly rejected it – a hospital job with no patient contact seemed unthinkable.

Perhaps a change within medicine? Maybe I could study public health? I was becoming increasingly interested in wider population issues and political advocacy. As a member of the International Physicians for the Prevention of Nuclear War I had come to like many of the people in community medicine. Their way of working seemed more cooperative and less hierarchical than that of many around me in surgery. I liked the idealism and sense of social justice. At medical school, public health had failed to stimulate me. In the 1970s, I had wanted to be a 'real' doctor who treated individual people, not faceless populations. I knew public health drove major benefits to health of the whole population. At the top of the cliff rather than the bottom. Was it too late to change?

After exploring the option of a change of specialty, I decided reducing my workload was more realistic. I stopped doing after-hours on-call work, took a pay cut and went off to fill a gap in the elective surgical service at Kenepuru Hospital. Reducing my workload made complete sense to me, but few surgeons went 'off call' as early. I was 53. I felt like an outlier letting the side down again, but a strong voice told me I had to change. At last I had started to listen to my body and act accordingly.

23.

A Late Awakening

IN THE 1970S, THERE WERE NO FEMALE orthopaedic surgeons in New Zealand. I'd never heard of one anywhere. My colleagues and I didn't give this much thought. If we had, I suspect we would have thought there was no place for women in orthopaedics.

This pervasive sexism was nothing new. When the medical school opened in Dunedin in 1875, all students were male. It remained like this for 16 years. In 1891, Emily Siedeberg was admitted, followed the next year by Margaret Cruickshank, but in the decades after few women followed them. By the time I entered medical school in 1964, women still made up only 12.5 percent of the class. Only 15 women were admitted that year.

From the start, men bullied, sexually harassed and discriminated against women in medicine. Even now, although women comprise most medical school entrants, they still have trouble breaking into male-dominated surgical specialties. This is especially true of orthopaedics. Today, only one in 20 New Zealand orthopaedic surgeons is female, and in Australia and the US the percentage is about the same.

My personal awakening came after I had operated on an accident victim named Jason. He was a 115-kilogram, heavily muscled man in his mid-20s whose motorbike had collided with a car at an intersection. He arrived at Middlemore Hospital's emergency department with a mild concussion and in tremendous pain. He had blanked out for several minutes but was now fully conscious. The ambulance staff had splinted his leg but hadn't given him strong painkillers as they didn't want to cloud his consciousness and prevent us assessing the severity of his head injury.

The department's house surgeon, Mark, confirmed the ambulance attendant's diagnosis of a broken femur and also suspected an elbow injury. He immediately set up an IV drip and sent a specimen of blood for cross-matching to allow for a possible blood transfusion. A patient with a fractured femur bleeds freely into the thigh. They can quickly lose 1000 to 1500 millilitres of blood, causing their blood pressure to fall. Most such patients need blood transfusion.

I was the orthopaedic registrar on call. I was just finishing operating on a patient when I received a message relayed by Zoe, the circulating nurse. (Circulating nurses remain unscrubbed, don't have to gown up, and can touch anything in the theatre except the scrubbed-up staff and the sterilised part of the patient. They can therefore answer the phone.)

'It's A&E,' Zoe said. 'They have a multi-trauma – motorbike versus car. KO'd, a bust femur and possibly elbow. They've set up a drip. They want you down there ASAP.'

'Oh dear,' I said, 'another Kawasaki.' We already had two young male motorcyclists with badly smashed femurs in traction on the ward. 'I hope this one is suitable for a K-rod.'

While Zoe held the phone to my ear I had a brief talk to the house surgeon. 'If his head is okay, give him 15 milligrams of morphine,' I said. 'Get the portable X-ray over and get films of the femur, including the knee on the affected side, the hip and whole pelvis, chest, head and affected elbow. Get blood off for crossmatch and order four units of blood. Put up a bag of plasma to support the circulation until the blood arrives. I'll be right down when I've sewn up here. Thanks, Mark.'

Blood and Bone

When I arrive at A&E, I check that Jason's airway is all right. His respiratory rate and pulse are raised, but he has good colour and his blood pressure is normal, indicating reasonable oxygenation and no shock.

His right leg is well immobilised in a splint. I ask him questions to assess his state of consciousness. He answers appropriately. I say, 'Do you have pain anywhere else besides your right leg?'

'Yes,' he says, 'my chest hurts when I breathe in. And my right elbow is sore.'

I systematically examine his body for signs of other injuries. I compress his chest and pelvis, palpate his abdomen, and examine his neck and all four limbs searching for tenderness.

I feel for pulses below his right thigh at knee and ankle, and below his right elbow at the wrist. I ask him to move his fingers and toes. I test the skin sensation of his foot and hand, looking for any vascular or neurological damage caused by fractures above.

We check his spine by 'log-rolling' his body.

We gently take off his splint. The leg below mid-thigh is rotated outwards at a grotesque angle. Using scissors, we cut through his leather trousers. I always hate the destruction of perfectly good clothing, including the elegant leathers worn by motorbikers, but conventional undressing causes too much disturbance at the fracture and may increase bleeding and pain.

The skin over the fracture is stretched by the bone ends, but there is no wound. The right elbow is swollen and there is a ragged deep wound full of road dirt. To minimise the chance of infection it will need antibiotics now, and a thorough clean-up in the theatre to remove damaged and contaminated tissue. 'Stick a gram of flucloxacillin into the drip please,' I say.

The X-rays show a fracture of the femur. Thankfully, it is suitable for a rod. When I trained, the operation for cleanly broken, mainly transverse fractures of the thigh bone was called 'rodding of the femur'. In the 1970s we used a rod called the Küntscher nail, named for the German surgeon who devised the technique.

A house surgeon, Janet, is helping me. Ann is the scrub nurse. 'Knife please, Ann,' I say. I open the fracture site with a 12-centimetre incision, cutting down through subcutaneous fat to expose the ends of the bone. There is a ragged hole through the full thickness of the quadriceps muscle where the sharp broken ends of the femur have penetrated.

I tell Janet, 'When we operate on a bone, we have to make sure we don't harm vital nerves and blood vessels on the way in. Get down to bone and stay there.' It's the safety mantra we all chant.

I ask Ann for the saline syringe and wash away small

fragments of bone, trying to disturb as little as possible the outside soft tissue covering of the bone, the periosteum.

I grab the bone ends of the femur with large forceps and use all my strength to stretch them out to their full length, overcoming the pull of the muscles. 'Bloody hell,' I say, 'this guy's muscle is like the one in the chimp's arm we fixed up at the zoo the other day.' (I had helped a vet drain a bone infection caused by a bite and been amazed by the size of the chimp's muscles.)

While maintaining the pull, I increase the bend in the bone ends and manipulate one bone end onto the other, fitting the jagged ends together like a jigsaw. I then ask Janet to grab the bone-holders and hold the bone fragments in line while I fire the rod down to her. I make an incision at the top of the femur, over the bony lump we all have where our hip girth is measured. Through this incision I penetrate the top of the bone with a sharp spike, or awl, then pass a stout guide wire through the marrow of the two main bone fragments. Over the top of the wire, I feed a hollow drill. This allows me to widen the bone canals to the width of the nail we will use to fix the two fragments together.

Then another strong-man act: I hammer the hollow nail over the guide wire. The nail is about the thickness of a little finger, but of a diameter and length to fit the widened bone canal perfectly. The fit is tight, so I have to hammer hard. The nail moves across the fracture. We see from the X-ray taken by the radiographer that the length and line of the femur are back to normal.

That night over dinner I relate my day's work to Pamela. I tell her that Janet, my house surgeon, was a great help in the operation. 'Why are there no women orthopaedic surgeons then?' she says in an accusatory tone. I explain that the operation involved fixing a broken femur on a 115-kilogram man. 'It took all my strength,' I say. 'I don't think there'd be many women able to do an operation like that.'

Pamela is not impressed. 'I don't see that as a problem. Some women will be strong enough. If they're not, all they'd need to do is to get a male in to assist. There must be strong men available to assist with that part of the operation under instruction.'

Her words stuck with me. She was right: there were male house surgeons, registrars or nurses whom a female registrar or surgeon might use to help with the heavy stuff – if necessary. Soon after this, technology was developed that made physical strength much less necessary. Modern power tools made for lighter work, especially for operations such as hip replacements. Most women were easily strong enough. But there was to be no female orthopaedic surgeon or trainee in New Zealand for another decade.

After the late '70s, the treatment of fractured lower limb long bones changed completely with the introduction of a portable X-ray system that could be turned around the body part, projecting the image from all angles onto a TV monitor. Heaving bones out to length by opening the thigh, grabbing and yanking them was now superfluous. With the help of the image intensifier the surgeon could treat most fractures of the femur, including those badly smashed into pieces, with a minimally invasive operation.

A major advantage was not having to expose the fracture site. Most fractures are 'closed': there is no breach in the skin. No matter what precautions are taken, making an incision through soft tissues to put bone fragments back together again risks introducing the much-feared infection of the bone, osteomyelitis. Before antibiotics, many patients with open fractures – ones where the skin was broken – died from overwhelming infection of the bone, which spread through the body. Military surgeons amputated limbs with open fractures because of this dreaded complication.

Not long before operating on Jason, I had tackled the same thing with Brent, a 22-year-old plumber who had also been involved in a motorbike crash. A week after the surgery, Brent's thigh wound had become red, hot and swollen. 'My thigh hurts like hell and I feel really crook,' he told me. 'I'm cold and shivery even though the nurse says I have a temperature.'

A Late Awakening

It was obvious he had a severe infection. When we opened his wound, it was full of pus. We irrigated the site with saline and removed the infected material. Then we left a tube open to the outside to allow further drainage and poured antibiotics into his drip.

The fracture refused to unite. Three more operations took place: one to get bone shavings from his pelvis, another to pack these around his fractured femur, and much later, when his bone eventually healed, to remove the metal rod and so reduce the chances of another infection flaring up. By the time he returned to work 16 months later, he had had a total of five operations and nearly required a sixth to free up his stiff knee. His quad muscles had become stuck fast to the healing fracture. He spent months with physios before achieving enough flexibility in his knee to allow him to return to his plumbing job, where he had to bend and crouch.

The closed technique has made this kind of disaster much less likely. Now, to line up broken fragments of a fractured femur, the surgeon passes a steel pin across the upper tibia (the shin bone) or lower femur and attaches a steel hoop to the two ends protruding outside the skin. A string is attached to the hoop and fed onto a ratchet with a handle at the lower end of the operating table. By turning this handle downwards, the surgeon pulls the limb out to its full length. There's no need for brute force:

a reasonably strong child could do this.

Using the X-ray machine to check progress, the surgeon then passes screws through the femur and rod, above and below the fracture, through small stab skin incisions. This stabilises the rod in the bone and prevents later shortening. Surgeons, female and male, can successfully treat badly smashed long bones with multiple fragments this way.

With these technical advances, women began putting up their hands to become trainees. I was glad about this: I had come to see no reason to deny half the population the opportunity to take up orthopaedics. In October 2020 the European Federation of National Associations of Orthopaedics and Traumatology stated that the critical mass for effective diversity is 30 percent. Their global survey showed no country had yet achieved this percentage of women in orthopaedics. Estonia topped the list with 27 percent. Various countries followed: UK eleven percent; US 6.1 percent, New Zealand 5.1 percent and Australia 4.3 percent. However, in 2021 New Zealand's trainee intake jumped to 25% female. The Australian figures are also climbing.

My experience is that in general women make more caring doctors than men; they are more sensitive to their patients' needs and more conscientious in their work. Their surgery is just as good. There is science to back this up: comparative studies on mortality rates and other measures

A Late Awakening

of surgical success show that women equal or better their male counterparts. Most patients express no gender preference for their surgeon.

When I was teaching fifth-year students musculoskeletal medicine and orthopaedics, I would tell them that most of New Zealand's graduating doctors were female but only about five percent of orthopaedic surgeons. I was curious to discover why they thought so few women took up the specialty. Some mentioned the unhealthy work style with little time off for relaxation, others the strongly competitive atmosphere. But most blamed the dominant male culture. Many women didn't see a job involving the use of hammers, drills and saws – 'toys for the boys' – as appealing. These stereotypes have been shaped by a culture where boys were taught woodwork and girls cooking and sewing.

Things are changing. School children of both sexes now learn a range of skills. Women are moving into carpentry, the construction industry and other trades. And in orthopaedics, discrimination is waning. Grace, who recently finished her five-year training, told me, 'I can't say I have been treated differently or unfairly. From my initial exposure to orthopaedics as a fourth-year medical student right through to fellowship and across eight district health boards, I have not felt discriminated against.'

Just as Pamela suggested 45 years ago, Grace calls for some 'muscle' when she needs it. 'I have used male scrub nurses and theatre orderlies to assist me in operations. Most are excited to be asked and some are nervous, but I always explain that whatever they are doing – for example, holding the pelvis down while I pull a hip in, or pulling a leg in a certain way – is under my instruction. I have never been ashamed to use men in this way.'

Grace said women are much more likely than men to be reserved and proceed with caution. 'They will say they have never done x procedure before, whereas the men will just wing it.'

A problem women cited was the inflexibility of surgical training programmes: this had discouraged them from taking time off for childbearing and childcare. In a questionnaire one surgical trainee, Isabel, said, 'If you take time off to have children, people perceive that your brain also fell out of your vagina and you have to start again from the beginning.'

But there's hope. Emma, a recent orthopaedic trainee wrote: 'Regarding pregnancy in training, there has been a huge change recently. It used to be that if a trainee missed six weeks of a six-month run, the run would not count and had to be made up later. Hence, some of us planned for babies to arrive near or around the end of a run. This has now been changed to pro rata: time done is time counted.'

Grace, who entered the training scheme in 2009, said, 'I think things have changed in the ten years since. I remember feeling a sense of dread, and quite honestly fear, as the first woman pregnant during the training. However, over subsequent years I have had some positive comments and seem to have started a trend among the female trainees, with several doing the same.'

Recently, operations performed by all New Zealand general surgical trainees from 2012 to 2017 were investigated. The results showed that female trainees were the primary operator in fewer cases than their male counterparts. One of the study's authors, Associate Professor Elizabeth Dennett, said this didn't surprise her. 'There's an old surgical maxim: See one, do one, teach one. And there used to be a joke among female trainees: see a hundred, do a hundred, then maybe teach one. Women tend to be more reticent about their abilities. If they're not, they're labelled as bolshie or premenstrual, whereas men are being "affirmative".

'There is also a "chicken and egg" phenomenon at play. The supervisor may perceive reticence as a lack of confidence and decide to take over the operation, which makes the trainee feel she isn't competent.'

The reticence of women about their abilities has shown up in other research. Women are more likely to suffer from 'imposter syndrome', a psychological pattern in which they doubt their accomplishments and have a persistent, often internalised fear of being exposed as a fraud. It is characterised by perfectionism, overworking, undermining one's own achievements, fear of failure and discounting praise.

Over a hundred years ago, some men objected to women pursuing higher education at all, claiming it would weaken their constitution, which was best suited for childbearing and caring for their family. Truby King, who founded the Plunket Society, argued that higher education placed too great a strain on women's lives and was thus detrimental to the vitality of the race. Doctors like King would likely have serious heart trouble should they be able to see the medical classes I have lectured, where around 55 percent of the students are women.

Many medical school lecturers argued that 'women medicals' (as they were known) were denying men a place at medical school and would likely marry, have children and leave the profession. The theory was initially borne out: of the first 50 female graduates, 30 married and gave up medicine. One reason was no doubt the disapproval of these pillars of the establishment. Women had difficulty finding employment after graduation; those employing young doctors preferred to hire men like themselves.

Having gained entrance to medical school, women still had hurdles to jump. Teachers were troubled dealing with the anatomy of genitals. Historian Dorothy Page would write: 'Professor [of Anatomy] Scott asked Emily

A Late Awakening

Siedeberg to absent herself from two of his anatomy classes … he taught her separately.'

A woman student graduating in 1903 noted that 'the lecturer on public health and medical jurisprudence once stopped in the middle of a class and said to two women, "Now I come to the part of my lecture that I refuse to give before women. Therefore, the women leave the room or I will leave it." Covered with confusion and accompanied by the hoots and jeers of their fellow students, the women left the class.'

Some prominent teachers behaved towards female students in a manner that now seems hardly credible. My distant relative Eefie White was one of them. Dorothy Page quotes one of his students Barbara Heslop, who later became professor of pathology at Otago Medical School: 'Eefie White … would often ask one member of the class to come out to the front with him during a lecture or clinic. If he chose a girl, he would conduct most of the class with his arm around her waist. … Medicine was still very much a "gentlemen's club" whose members tolerated us.'

Although teachers may have been merely disapproving of or patronising to female students, male colleagues could be openly hostile. In classes, as elsewhere in the university, segregation was the norm. The women sat in the front row. Dorothy Page recounts that 'in one course the women regularly found themselves under painful attack from male students with peashooters … until the day the women all arrived early and sat in the back row. On this occasion the men were generous enough to applaud, but if women came in late or gave a stupid answer they hooted and catcalled. …

'In 1920, members of the Otago Medical Students Association made it very clear that they were not wanted. One speaker referred to "a matter of sex antipathy" and complained that "everywhere women were invading men's rights".'

Subsequently the Association voted to exclude women, arguing that, as the women numbered at least 50, they should form their own association.

There was disrespect towards cadavers. Dorothy Page reports 'male students … running down the stairs, brandishing an arm or leg. … Emily Siedeberg had a very unpleasant time with her classmates. They did not want lady doctors. … the young men would throw the flesh at her at every chance they got.'

Although this flesh throwing seems to have reigned only in the early days of the medical school, sexual innuendo towards women persisted. Robin Briant, in 1984 elected the first woman doctor member and later chair of the New Zealand Medical Council from 1990 to 1996, comments on her experiences in the mid-1960s in *The Early Medical Women of New Zealand* edited by Cindy Farquar.

A Late Awakening

'The anatomy tutors who wandered around amongst the cadavers and the students – some of them were particularly sexist. ... there were one or two notoriously unpleasant people – not so much putting down, as just being plain sexually rude and suggestive.'

I witnessed and was appalled by blatant examples of misogyny during my clinical years at medical school. Even before my classmates and I had met a particular professor, we had heard of his sexist comments. I personally saw him baiting my female classmates and had worse reported to me. One male colleague of mine saw him come up to the front row, where the women often sat, and pronounce, 'You ladies will never become orthopaedic surgeons: you're not strong enough. And, oh, you'll probably never marry, unless it's to one of your classmates.'

I have learnt that other senior orthopaedic surgeons also made condescending remarks to potential and established female trainees, and even to women who had fully trained and gained their fellowship.

Trying to understand this overt sexism and whether it still exists, I recently contacted several women, including those I had worked with when they were trainees. Amelia, a house surgeon, told me she was keen to take up orthopaedics but nobody was interested. 'I am 161 centimetres tall and Asian,' she wrote. 'On my orthopaedics run I was coming to work an hour early and staying behind late to assist in theatre. I would go to theatres on weekends and most nights. I had been told many times before that I looked the "dermatology type". Comments like "you're just weak" and "your hands are too small" were routine. What they don't know is that I grew up on a farm with ponies, played rugby and soccer all the way through school, went to Everest base camp.'

Emma wrote: 'Four girls (all trainees) going through one training centre got the "orthopaedics is not for girls". We were told to consider dermatology. One of them got, "You're a lovely girl but would be more suited to radiology or pathology." I got summoned by a consultant, sat down and told, "Girls don't have enough testosterone. You don't have as much strength, and you need strength in orthopaedics. You will have children and your children need you. You can't be a good doctor and a good mother at the same time".'

Even after they graduated as orthopaedic surgeons, the women were subjected to insults from senior male colleagues. After passing her final exam, while socialising with the examiners and drinking the traditional sherry, Meg was told, 'Of course, women in orthopaedics lower its status.'

I worked with Olive when she was a junior in the operating theatre. She told me a story. 'Having just passed the fellowship exam we were at an orthopaedic dinner. A well-known orthopod approached us, introduced himself and said something along the lines of, "I guess I need to congratulate you girls on becoming surgeons. I'm going to follow with interest what happens to you. I'm not sure I agree with you having been trained at all; I had no idea New Zealand was so short of hand surgeons. But at any rate you should come over here and meet my wife. She trained as a doctor, never worked a day in her life".'

Karen Smith, the first female orthopaedic surgeon in Australasia, entered the training programme in 1983 and is today a hand surgeon at Middlemore Hospital and in private practice in Auckland. She has a partner and two children. She told her story in Dr Rosy Fenwicke's book *In Practice: The lives of New Zealand women doctors in the 21st century*, published in 2004. At the age of 15 Karen decided 'with light-bulb-like clarity' to become a doctor. She immediately struck opposition. 'My family GP promptly attempted to change my mind. He told me I would never marry, never have children. Medicine was not the place for women.'

After a month working on an orthopaedic run, Karen chose to specialise. 'The obvious practicality and immediacy of results appealed to me. Broken bones were fixed, crippled limbs were straightened. Pain, deformity and suffering were healed. …

'At my interview for basic surgical training, one general surgeon actually laughed outright at the preposterousness of my ambition.'

Karen pressed on. She was generally accepted by her male colleagues but 'never felt the same as the other surgical trainees. I'm not referring to the bluff, sweaty changing-room male bonhomie, but rather to their attitude, their confidence and their almost instinctive superiority. When things got tough … and things in the operating theatre turned to custard, my male colleagues would rise above it, apparently unshaken, their mana intact. They were the great colossus, the male orthopaedic registrars, striding onward past the wrecks of a few disasters.'

Males like me have felt a little less confident, but we certainly didn't show it. Nor did we talk about it. Admit weakness? Not likely. We hardened up, bluffed, tried to look cool.

Karen outlined some of the serious problems for female graduates from the orthopaedic training scheme. They often had difficulty obtaining a job in a public hospital. Male colleagues excluded them from jobs in private practice or audits of cases, a necessary collegial activity to maintain a practising certificate from the New Zealand Medical Council. There was 'blokeish teasing' and irritating banter such as 'must have slept with the prof to get on the training scheme'. A female orthopaedic surgeon pointed to a recent Auckland orthopaedic conference dinner invitation: '19.00 p.m. – Registrar Graduation Dinner. Northern Club with wives.'

Karen didn't let the setbacks and put-downs deter her. 'There was no way I was ever going to ask for help. I battled on.'

Sue Stott entered orthopaedic training a year after Karen. She is now professor of paediatric orthopaedic surgery at Auckland University, with interests in chronic physical disability in children. Early in her career Sue was registrar for orthopaedic surgeon Richard Nicol. She recalled, 'The training committee made a point of phoning Richard to let him know he would be having two female registrars [and] as the first two women on the scheme we would need to be treated differently. ... Richard surprised them by saying he saw female trainees as no different to male trainees and would treat us exactly the same, something to his credit he absolutely did.'

Margy Pohl, a Whangarei orthopaedic surgeon, has front-footed a new organisation, LIONZ – Ladies In Orthopaedics New Zealand. The group runs courses, including sawbone workshops, for female medical students around the country. These workshops are the way today's orthopaedic surgeons learn some vital operations.

When I was training, we learnt on the job: our sawbones were real bones. Inevitably we made errors on our patients. I shudder at the memory. The 'bones' in the sawbone workshops are replicas of hard plastic. The operator can safely cut, drill, screw, apply metal plates and wires and insert rods or prosthetic joints. Mock-ups of knees and other joints allow learners to practise without the bleeding that can obscure vision and the need to hurry through an operation to minimise the time the patient is anaesthetised.

As a lecturer I was once surprised by a female student. During a lesson, we were discussing the technique of aspirating a knee joint to draw off fluid. This is sometimes necessary to relieve pain, or to test an effusion in an inflamed but non-traumatised knee in order to make a diagnosis about the type of arthritis – rheumatoid, gout, sepsis, etc. After describing where best to insert the needle, I said, 'Sometimes there's a lot of clot in the fluid, so to prevent blockage you'll need to use a wide-gauge needle – something like a number 15 or broader. That's about the thickness of a standard pen refill, and two to three times the outside diameter of the usual needle for skin injections. Do you think we should put local anaesthetic into the skin first?'

The student's hand shot up. 'Nah,' she said, 'just ask the patient to man up.'

24.

Union Man

AFTER 27 YEARS AS A CONSULTANT, I resigned from Wellington Hospital. I was in my early sixties and it felt right to scale down. I was increasingly concerned by the climate change crisis and was becoming involved in political advocacy. I had joined Ora Taiao: The New Zealand Climate and Health Council, an organisation of medical professionals working to make the public and politicians aware of the threats climate disruption poses to human health and urging rapid action. As with Physicians against Nuclear War, I have learnt much from the highly motivated doctors in this group. As a climate change action advocate I have lectured to medical and community groups. I belong to transport groups promoting climate-friendly choices for Wellington city.

I also furthered my love of teaching, taking up a part-time job as coordinator of the musculoskeletal course for fifth-year medical students at the medical school campus in Wellington. A colleague and I demonstrated to and supervised students as they learned techniques to elicit the signs of dysfunction of joints, muscles and tendons. Sometimes we used professional actors. Circa Theatre's Ross Jolly became an expert 'patient'. I asked him to give feed-back to the students on their examination technique, 'Some of you grabbed my joint far too roughly,' he admonished the students one day. 'If I'd been sore, you'd have made me scream. No way I'd come back to see you.'

I continued this teaching for nine years, combining it with a half-day a week of private practice. The work was enjoyable and I felt rewarded. However, my cosy teaching arrangement ended abruptly. In early 2015 the head of department at the medical school asked about my plans. I told him I was enjoying teaching, feedback from the students was good and I wanted to continue. I believed we had verbally agreed I would work for at least another two years. However, at the end of the academic year, when the students had dispersed, he bluntly informed me, 'We don't need you next year.'

I had been more of a thorn in his side than I realised.

Union Man

I had become concerned that undergraduate students' exposure to orthopaedics – and more generally musculoskeletal medicine – was low compared with their exposure to general surgery and other specialties. Research has shown that musculoskeletal is the second most common condition with which patients present to New Zealand GPs; it makes up about 20 percent of their work. Furthermore, work done in 2009 had estimated that such disorders cost New Zealand more than ten billion dollars a year. There was, therefore, a discrepancy between the teaching time allocated to these conditions and what family doctors needed to know.

In 2010 I had assigned a fifth-year medical student, Megan Brown, to carry out a study of trainee GPs graduating from the country's four medical schools. Megan's research showed that musculoskeletal teaching made up only 2.3 to 4 percent of the five-year undergraduate curriculum. In a questionnaire Megan had asked the trainee GPs whether this had equipped them adequately for their work in general practice. Nearly half said the training had been far too short. Of nine simple skills, they felt underprepared in six.

The questionnaire had arrived near exam time so only a third of the doctors responded, which made the conclusions statistically deficient. Even so, I thought they justified trying to improve the situation. I engaged in head-banging, approaching the dean of the medical school and others. I came up against an entrenched academic hierarchy with no appetite for change. I was told by one, 'Oh, teachers in every specialty want more teaching time.' The university was also on an economy drive. I became tired of my boss's often repeated cry, 'How many times do I have to tell you that the university has no money?'

My enquiries since have revealed little if any progress. Musculoskeletal conditions seldom kill people, which may account for the low teaching priority given them. But fixing them can greatly enhance a person's quality of life.

On top of pushing for more teaching time for musculoskeletal, I wanted to expand the teaching using actual patients. Hospital doctors are permitted to do this if the patients are fully informed and agree to being questioned and examined by medical students. 'Slow' clinics give students one-on-one access to patients who are attending hospital clinics for initial assessment. The clinics are 'slow' because extra time is required – 45 minutes instead of the usual 30.

These clinics had been used by a colleague at Hutt Hospital for years and feedback from students showed they were popular. With student numbers increasing, doctors were finding it increasingly difficult to give students enough clinical teaching time in public hospitals. My plan would have required minimal financial input, with any costs shared by the hospital and the university.

I made preliminary arrangements with my hospital colleagues and the administration, but my university boss was sceptical. He objected to my approaching the hospital hierarchy and my colleagues without consulting him. An academic with strong research credentials he did not have a medical degree. Despite that, he had been put in charge of the Department of Surgery and Anaesthesia. Not surprisingly, he had little understanding of the needs of medical students.

Nor, it seemed, did the dean of the medical school, a former practising psychiatrist. She informed me, 'Medical students are so bright these days they can mainly learn the skills needed in your department online.' I was flabbergasted that she thought it reasonable to replace me with a computer. Videos and online lessons are useful, but practical clinical skills are best taught hands-on, with instruction and supervision by experienced medical clinicians.

The advertisement for my replacement simply stated: 'We are looking for clinical experience in an area involving musculoskeletal medicine.' Good so far, I thought. But it went on 'and a relevant qualification in an area of health care (e.g. nursing, physiotherapy, paramedicine).' It seemed they no longer wanted a doctor to teach students studying to become doctors. Not only that, the successful applicant would have to obtain 'research funding and/or grants from industry'. I was being asked to leave because my teaching as an experienced clinician was not deemed enough. Research (I had done plenty on patients) was seen as most important.

To me, the advertisement signalled an attempt to downplay an important area of general practice, which is where the largest proportion of graduating doctors choose to work. A Medical Council workforce survey in 2018 showed that GPs made up over 57 percent of practising doctors, more than three times the next most numerous group, doctors practising internal medicine.

Since the mid '80s I had seen the introduction of what has been called 'managerialism' in hospitals – a shift in power from clinicians to managers, and a concern with budgetary efficiency over quality of patient care. When I was chair of the hospital's division of surgery, a former high-ranking manager of recently privatised Telecom was appointed CEO of the hospital. At Telecom, we learnt, he had been known as Chainsaw because of the swathe he cut through the staff employed there. He had no special knowledge of how hospitals and surgery worked. We called him Fretsaw. The move to managerialism made many experienced clinicians frustrated: we believed it hurt both patients and students.

Union Man

A couple of years before my teaching job was abruptly terminated, I had met a colleague in the lift. 'Coming to the drinks downstairs put on by the union?' she'd said cheerfully.

'Oh, what union is that?' I said. 'I didn't know we university teachers had one.'

I seldom turn down a social occasion, particularly around a few drinks, and I'm glad I didn't this time. I emerged a signed-up union man.

As soon as I was informed of my summary dismissal, I contacted my union representative. He arranged a meeting with my employer's human resources team and a professional mediator. It was deemed that since I had been employed for nine years as a teacher, even though on a yearly renewable contract, I was entitled to the equivalent conditions of a full-time employee. The result was that I gained compensation.

I had noted as an aside that after nine years, my employer hadn't even farewelled me with the customary morning tea. A bit small-minded I have since thought, but I felt humiliated at the time. The mediator asked, 'Well, do you want one?' After I exclaimed that I would probably choke on my muffin, my union rep persuaded me, 'Go on, we'll get you a farewell.' I invited along some close colleagues. My previous boss had to say nice things about me. The muffins were delicious; I swallowed them easily.

Blood and Bone

For the next five years I ran a weekly fracture clinic at Kenepuru Hospital's accident and medical service, close to where I first developed the exciting new knee surgery techniques I learnt in Toronto. Thirty years later the small hospital still had the same friendly atmosphere and congenial work colleagues with whom I really enjoyed working. Many of my patients were needy and would otherwise have to travel 25 kilometres or so to Wellington Hospital. It felt well worthwhile.

It was a pleasant journey as I rode my bike 10kms across the city to the railway station and took the train, followed by a short walk to the hospital. Working only half days, I no longer felt the need to go for a jog around the hospital grounds to relieve stress. This was just as well as my knees and hips were wearing out. Biking a great substitute.

Many of the simple fractures I treated were in children. In the growing child, bone heals about twice as quickly as it does in adults. So called 'green-stick fractures', where a bone is buckled or bent without fracturing right through, are common.

I got a lot of kudos for removing plaster-of-Paris casts from children who'd suffered mild green stick fractures around the wrist. Many just needed a splint, and this could be easily removed to allow the skin to be washed. When I removed the plaster cast from six-year-old Jimmy his mother said, 'That's such a relief. Jimmy complains of the itchiness and the smell.' I heard this often.

Some parents see plaster as the only cure for a fracture and worry that the broken bone will move out of place without it. I reassure them that splints are perfectly adequate for stable fractures in young children. 'We're just treating the pain. The slight bend in the arm will remodel with growth. Most will entirely straighten out. Later in life many kids don't even remember which arm was broken.'

I loved following up these children after their simple injuries. By the time I saw them a week or two later most were in little or no pain. I liked to have fun with them.

The orthopaedics was easy but the computerisation of medical records, the forms I had to fill out to order investigations and treatments or sign off patients from work, caused me headaches. My nurse colleagues were a generation younger. 'Tina,' I yelp, 'help! I can't get into this bloody programme.'

'Oh,' she says patiently, 'you have to change your password every six weeks.'

'What on earth for?'

'Security.'

Most of the rolling farmland and groves of trees that surrounded the hospital 35 years ago are no more. The old Porirua Hospital grounds, gained by Ngāti Toa in a Treaty of Waitangi settlement, are being used for much-needed accommodation. The maternity hospital, where a colleague and I had examined newborns for congenital musculoskeletal abnormalities, has been replaced with a car park. A huge concrete flyover is being built; it will link the new Transmission Gully motorway with the road in front of the hospital. Many people see this as progress. I'm less sure.

Today the intense drama of the operating theatre is just a memory. I no longer cut patients' soft tissues to rearrange them or to gain access to their skeletons so I can straighten and fix their broken bones or worn joints. I do not peer via scope and camera at a screen to manipulate their joint structures with fine instruments. There are no more heroics on the operating theatre stage, and no more anxiety as I climb into bed at night wondering if I'll be called to handle an emergency. It is enough.

Acknowledgements

Thanks to all my senior medical colleagues who passed on their wisdom. Particularly my close mentor, Bill Gillespie who also showed his faith in me when I most needed it. My older brother Garnet Tregonning for his example from childhood, his generous help when we worked closely together on the same orthopaedic team, and his encouragement all through my career. John Bartlett, who generously hosted me in Melbourne, Australia, passing on valuable tips on surgical technique. To Robin Briant for her review of the script and generous endorsement.

To other close colleagues: Tim Astley, Grant Kiddle and Tim Gregg for reading the script and for helpful comment. Andrew Spiers for his insights on modern anaesthesia and Jane Outrimm for searching my past clinical records for some of the patient stories.

My female orthopaedic colleagues for relating their experiences.

Surgery is a team effort: thanks to the unfailing

help and support from my nursing colleagues. Also from my junior medical and other health worker colleagues. To Louise Goossens, medical photographer for her expertise, she not only provided the image for the book cover, but also created many of the images in the photo section. All my patients: they teach us doctors about their conditions if we will listen.

My medical school classmates: Rae Varcoe for permission to quote her poem 'Cadaver Spoken Here' from her book *Tributary*. My close classmate friends – John Hutton for his support during my career, reading the script and helpful comment. Roger Mee my close fellow surgical trainee for editorial help.

Roger Robinson for permission to use his material from *PodiumRunner* and *Runner's World* magazines, and his publicised gratitude for his knee replacement (which he called 'Russell'). Elizabeth Dennet for sharing conclusions from her co-authored research on autonomy in operations among female and male general surgical trainees. Dorothy Page for permission to use excerpts from her book: *Anatomy of a Medical School: A History of Medicine at the University of Otago*. Rosy Fenwicke for excerpts from her book: *The Lives of New Zealand Women Doctors in the 21st Century*. Grant Nisbett read the script, made comment and generously allowed me to name a piece of our surgical hardware the 'Nisbo'. To Neale Pitches and

Acknowledgements

Mary O'Regan who read the script and made constructive comment. To other experts who read and endorsed the script: Nicky Hager, Brian Turner, and Grahame Sydney.

My actor son Mark Tregonning stimulated me to describe the drama in the operating theatre, comparing it to that on the stage. He has encouraged me all through my writing and also gave me his insightful help with the script. My friend, Mary Varnham at Awa Press having stimulated me to write this book then suggested its title and expertly edited it over many hours. Her alchemy has transformed the book.

Thanks to actor, director and writer Ross Jolly for being a model 'patient/lecturer'. To Kenepuru Hospital receptionist Hine Simpson for information about old Porirua psychiatric hospital treatments.

My thanks to my publisher Brett Cross of Atuanui Press for his expertise, attention to detail and excellent communication. And to Diane Lowther for her final review of the script.

My choice of career has, at times, made for a difficult journey for my wife Pamela; through it all she has lovingly supported me, and been my rock.

To all of these: sine qua non.